STROKE EXPLAINED

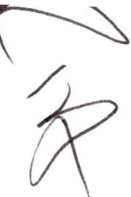

Provided as a service to medicine by 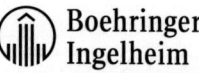 Boehringer Ingelheim

STROKE EXPLAINED

Ronald S MacWalter BMSc(Hons) MD FRCP(Edin) FRCP(Glas)
Consultant Physician and Honorary Senior Lecturer,
Stroke Studies Centre, Department of Medicine,
Ninewells Hospital and Medical School, Dundee

Hazel W Fraser RGN
Stroke Coordinator,
NHS Fife Acute Hospitals Trust,
Queen Margaret Hospital,
Dunfermline, Fife, Scotland

ALTMAN

Published by Altman Publishing, 7 Ash Copse, Bricket Wood, St Albans, Herts, AL2 3YA, England

First edition 2003

© 2003 Ronald S MacWalter and Hazel W Fraser

The rights of Ronald S MacWalter and Hazel W Fraser to be identified as Authors of this Work have been asserted by them in accordance with the Copyright, Designs and Patents Act 1988.

Typeset in 10/12.5 Optima by Scribe Design, Gillingham, Kent
Printed in Great Britain by George Over Ltd, Rugby

ISBN 1 86036 022 X

All rights reserved. No part of this publication may be reproduced, stored in a retrieval system or transmitted in any form or by any means, electronic, mechanical, photocopying, recording or otherwise, without the prior written permission of the publisher. Applications for permission should be addressed to the publisher at the address printed on this page.

The publisher makes no representation, express or implied, with regard to the accuracy of the information contained in this book and cannot accept any legal responsibility or liability for any errors or omissions that may be made.

A catalogue record for this book is available from the British Library

∞ Printed on acid-free text paper, manufactured in accordance with ANSI/NISO Z39.48-1992 (Permanence of Paper)

CONTENTS

About the authors	vii
Foreword	ix
1 Introduction	1
2 What is a stroke?	3
3 Causes and risk factors	7
4 What are the symptoms of a stroke?	19
5 How is a stroke diagnosed?	27
6 The ideal consultation – what should I tell my doctor?	37
7 What treatments are available?	39
8 Recovery and complications	47
9 Frequently asked questions	55
10 Case studies	59
Appendix	67
Index	71

ABOUT THE AUTHORS

Ronald MacWalter is a Consultant Physician in General Medicine and Acute Stroke Medicine at Ninewells Hospital and Medical School, Dundee, Scotland. His medical school training was at the University of Dundee Medical School and the University of Florida School of Medicine. He qualified in 1978. His post-graduate training in General Medicine and Stroke took place in Dundee and at the John Radcliffe Hospital, Oxford. He returned to Dundee in 1986 and set up the Stroke Studies Centre in the Department of Medicine. He runs an acute stroke unit in Ninewells Hospital and arranges the investigation and treatment of acute stroke patients and organizes rehabilitation services when required. He is involved with the establishment of a managed clinical network for stroke in Tayside.

Dr MacWalter's research interests include the causes of acute stroke and prognostic factors for recovery after acute stroke. He conducts collaborative research with other physicians, health psychologists and physiotherapists. He has lectured on stroke topics at many national and international meetings and has authored a number of papers and books on stroke and related topics. He has been heavily involved in the Scottish Intercollegiate Guideline Network (SIGN) guidelines on stroke and related topics. He is an executive committee member of the British Association of Stroke Physicians (BASP) and Scottish Heart and Arterial Risk Prevention Group (SHARP).

Hazel Fraser trained as a nurse at the predecessor of the University of Dundee School of Nursing. Coming back to work after raising a family, she moved into research medicine. She worked with Dr MacWalter in the Stroke Studies Centre for 10 years, combining research with practical help for stroke patients. She set up the Dundee Stroke Recovery Club with Dr MacWalter – this self-help group is affiliated to Chest, Heart & Stroke Scotland. In 2002 she started work as stroke coordinator for Fife, which involves developing stroke services across Fife, working with the multidisciplinary teams involved in stroke care, acting as a key contact for patients, carers and staff providing information, risk management and secondary prevention and education. She is particularly interested in patients' and carers' views of services provided and has presented her research findings at European and World Stroke conferences. She is a member of the SIGN Guideline group on management of dysphagia post-stroke and a committee member of the Scottish Stroke Nurse Forum. She holds a qualification in Counselling Skills and is currently studying for an MSc in Health Promotion.

FOREWORD

The study of stroke management still remains a 'Cinderella' subject, despite its importance in clinical medicine (stroke is the third commonest cause of death in Western countries).

This excellent volume will be widely acclaimed as it encapsulates an up-to-date account of stroke which ranges through aetiology, risk factors, clinical presentation and complications to treatments and rehabilitation. This is directed at a widely based audience which includes stroke sufferers and also covers a range of therapists, nurses and junior medical staff.

It is written in an easily read style and well illustrated with simple line diagrams, and CT and MRI images. It should be mandatory reading for all stroke patients and their families.

C D Forbes
MD FRCP FRSE
Professor of Medicine
Ninewells Hospital and Medical School, Dundee
and Chairman, Chest, Heart & Stroke Scotland

1 INTRODUCTION

When there's a problem, what people want most of all is information. This is especially true when the problem is a medical one. This book is one of a series, each one dealing with a particular medical condition. They are all written by expert doctors and health workers, so the information is accurate and up to date.

This particular book deals with stroke. It describes what a stroke is, how it is caused, who is at risk, what can be done to reduce the risks, and what can be done once a stroke has occurred. It has been written especially for patients, their families, and their carers, and although it is not meant to replace consultation with your own doctors and nurses, it will answer most of the questions you are likely to have and will provide a handy source of reference at all times.

2

2 WHAT IS A STROKE?

Stroke is a very serious illness. It is the brain equivalent of a heart attack. Some people call it a 'brain attack'. And it must be taken seriously. A stroke is as serious as a heart attack. Here are some basic facts about stroke.

- Stroke is the fourth commonest cause of death in the UK.
- Stroke is the leading cause of adult disability in the UK.
- Most people who experience a stroke survive.
- Most (approximately two-thirds) stroke survivors live in the community and are able to care for themselves.
- Strokes affect people of all ages.
- People under age 65 account for about a quarter of all strokes.
- Increasing age increases the chances of having a stroke.
- Positive lifestyle changes can reduce the chances of having a stroke.
- High blood pressure increases the chances of having a stroke and this can be treated efficiently nowadays.

Types of stroke

There are two types of stroke, both of which result in an interruption to the normal flow of blood within the brain. An ischaemic stroke (cerebral infarct) occurs when there is a blockage in an artery in the brain, perhaps caused by a blood clot. The word ischaemia relates to an interruption to blood flow. A haemorrhagic stroke (cerebral haemorrhage) occurs when there is bleeding from an artery in the brain, caused by a weak blood vessel bursting. The word haemorrhagic relates to blood loss.

Figures 2.1 and 2.2 show how a cerebral infarct and a cerebral haemorrhage damage the brain.

Computerized tomography (CT) scans are useful in confirming the diagnosis of stroke. Some CT scans showing normal images and different types of stroke are shown in Figures 2.3–2.5.

CT scans can differentiate a cerebral haemorrhage (Figure 2.4), which shows up as a dark (denser) area on the right side of the brain, from a

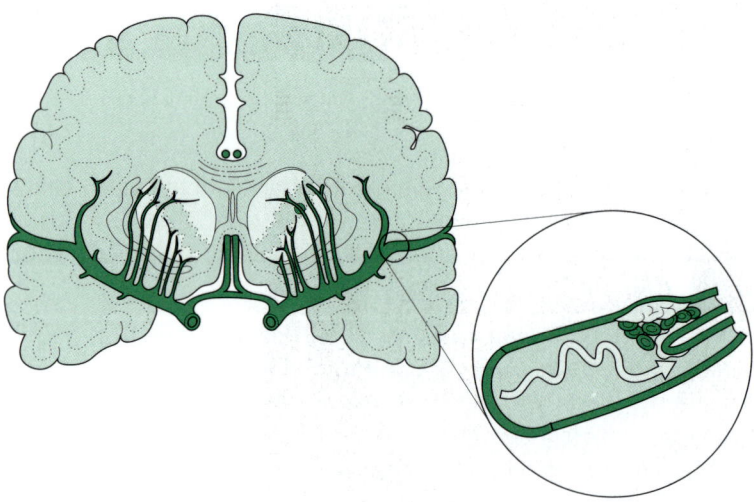

Figure 2.1 Ischaemic stroke can develop in two ways: disease (atherosclerosis) causes a thick, rough deposit to form on the inner wall of an artery, blocking the passageway or narrowing it, so that only a small amount of blood gets through; or a blood clot gets stuck in an artery and blocks the blood flow.

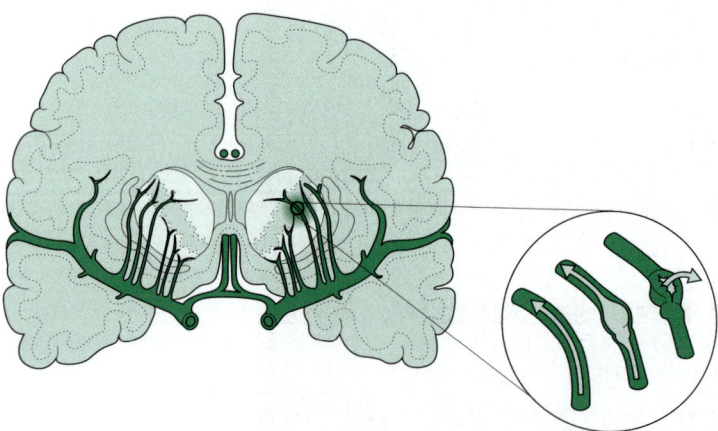

Figure 2.2 There are two types of haemorrhagic stroke: blood from a burst artery is forced into the tissue of the brain (intracerebral haemorrhage); or into the narrow space between the brain surface and the layer of tissue that covers the brain (subarachnoid haemorrhage).

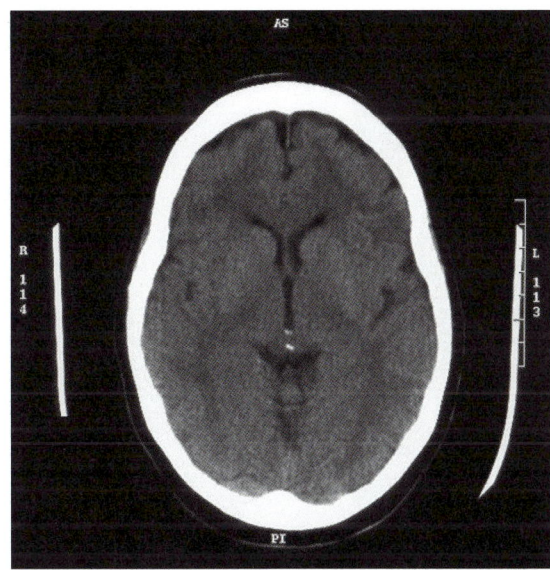

Figure 2.3 A normal CT scan.

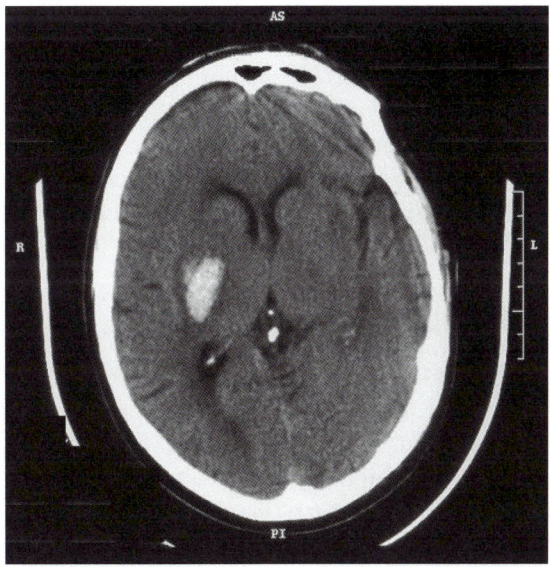

Figure 2.4 CT showing a cerebral haemorrhage.

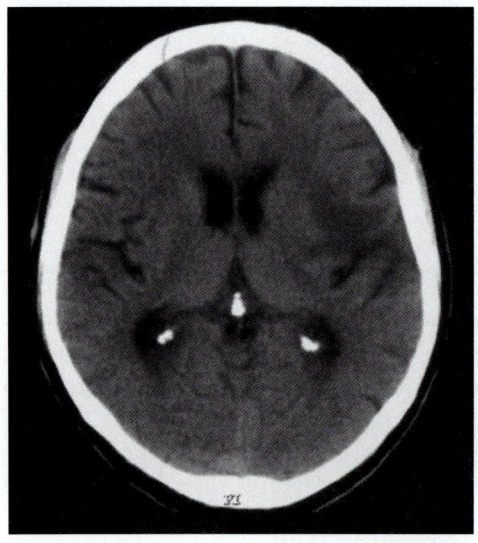

Figure 2.5 CT showing a cerebral infarct.

cerebral infarct (Figure 2.5) – this latter shows as a darker (less dense) area on the right side of the brain.

Transient ischaemic attacks (TIAs)

A transient ischaemic attack, TIA for short, is a sort of temporary minor stroke. It usually happens when a blood clot temporarily blocks an artery in the brain or neck. This prevents part of the brain getting the blood it needs, and this can result in some of the symptoms of a stroke. These episodes are transient, that is, temporary, and the blood clot soon moves on or dissolves away, and the effects disappear.

How common are strokes?

In fact, strokes and TIAs (or 'mini-strokes') are very common illnesses. Every year in the United Kingdom approximately 130 000 people have a stroke, although certain people are more likely to have a stroke than others. The good news is that there are some quite simple things that can be done to reduce the risk of having a stroke (see the section on lifestyle factors on page 9).

3 CAUSES AND RISK FACTORS

A stroke occurs when there is an interruption of blood flow in the brain. As described above, the interruption can be caused by a blocked artery (ischaemic stroke) or by a burst or leaking artery (haemorrhagic stroke). *Ischaemic* strokes are the most common and account for more than 80% of all strokes. *Haemorrhagic strokes* account for less than 20% of all strokes. Brain nerve cells are very sensitive to interruptions in their normal blood supply, and will die within minutes if they do not get blood. The location of the stroke within the brain affects the symptoms that are experienced.

Blocked blood vessels

Ischaemic strokes are the result of narrowing or clogging of arteries that supply the tissue of the brain, or by a blood clot or piece of debris breaking off from the heart or a blood vessel and causing one of the blood vessels leading to the brain to block.

Weak blood vessels

Haemorrhagic strokes are caused by an artery bursting and leaking blood into the brain. The force of blood into the brain tissue damages cells directly within the brain and also, by pressure effects, closes down other blood vessels supplying the brain. Sometimes this is due to a faulty artery with which the person has been born (a weakness in the artery wall which is then more susceptible to bursting – an aneurysm) or because the artery wall has become thin and brittle due to disease. Certain other conditions that make the clotting of blood a problem can also lead to a haemorrhagic stroke when there is relatively minor damage to the artery wall.

Risk factors that can increase the chances of stroke

Strokes usually occur because a combination of factors, such as certain medical conditions (e.g. high blood pressure), unhealthy lifestyle factors (e.g. smoking or poor diet) and inherited characteristics, come together. Strokes are seldom due to sudden shocks or arguments. Strokes are definitely not a punishment for bad deeds that people may have done.

There are basically two types of risk factors for most medical conditions. *Non-modifiable* risk factors are those that cannot be changed, such as one's age or sex. *Modifiable* risk factors, sometimes called *lifestyle factors*, are those that can be changed, such as smoking or being overweight.

Non-modifiable risk factors for stroke

- Age
- Gender
- Ethnic group
- Previous stroke
- Family history of stroke.

Age

Older people are at higher risk of a stroke than younger people. We all get older each day, and from the age of 55 onwards, the chances of having a stroke more than double every 10 years. This increase in risk with age happens relentlessly and dramatically. Therefore, older people must take great care to pay attention to those risk factors over which they have control.

Gender

Men are at risk at an earlier age than women. Therefore, at the same age, men will be at a slightly higher risk than women. Most stroke survivors tend to be women, however, because women generally live longer than men.

Ethnic group
Certain ethnic groups seem to be at higher risk. Afro-Caribbeans and people from the Indian subcontinent appear to have a higher risk of stroke. Afro-Caribbeans have high blood pressure more often than white people, which may be a contributory factor. People from the Far East have a higher risk of haemorrhagic stroke.

Previous stroke
Without appropriate treatment, the risk of another stroke in the 12 months after a first stroke is about one in ten. This is why a full investigation for potential causes and attention to all modifiable risk factors is so important after a stroke.

Family history
There is no doubt that some families have a higher risk of stroke than others. The risk of stroke is greater in people who have a family history of stroke and TIAs. It is important for such families to have risk factors identified and treated where possible, to reduce the risk of stroke.

Modifiable risk factors (lifestyle factors) for stroke
- Smoking
- Alcohol excess
- Diet and obesity
- Oral contraceptive pill
- Physical exercise.

Smoking
The risk of having a stroke is multiplied four times if you smoke. Blood vessels in your body constrict because of the chemicals and gases in tobacco smoke and this reduces blood flow. When this happens in vulnerable areas of the body like the brain, the blood is more likely to clot. So constricting the blood supply and promoting clotting are two ways in which smoking can make it more likely that a stroke will occur.

Stopping smoking will reduce your risks immediately. This will happen even if you have smoked for a very long time.

It is often very difficult to stop smoking. However, you can get help from clinics held locally, from nicotine replacement patches and gum, and from the use of some new drugs such as Zyban (bupropion). There is also a smoking phone helpline (see Appendix).

Alcohol

Drinking up to two small drinks of alcohol a day has been shown in studies to actually reduce the risk of stroke! The risk of stroke tends to increase after that, however. Heavy alcohol use will increase the risk of stroke dramatically, one reason being that it tends to increase blood pressure. As we have already seen, this can lead to the bursting of blood vessels.

Binge drinking is particularly unhealthy and this, together with regular heavy drinking, will increase the chances of having a stroke.

Diet and obesity

Obesity doubles the risk of developing high blood pressure, which is a major risk factor for stroke. Many doctors now measure obesity in terms of the body mass index (BMI). This is calculated from a person's weight in kilograms and height in metres by the following formula:

BMI = weight in kilograms divided by (height in metres)^2

For example, if a person weighs 10 stone 5 lb, this coverts into 145 lbs; 1 kg is equal to 2.2 lbs, so that 145 lbs = 65.9 kg. If the same person's height is 5 feet 8 inches, this converts into 68 inches; 1 inch is equal to 2.54 cm, so that 68 inches = 173 cm, or 1.73 metres. 1.73 squared (1.73 × 1.73) = 2.99. So, the BMI is given by 65.9 divided by 2.99, which equals 22.0.

This may seem a difficult calculation when described in words but it is actually very straightforward. Tables and graphs exist which allow you to read off your BMI from your weight and height (Figure 3.1), and your doctor or nurse may be able to give you one of these.

A normal healthy person of the correct weight for their height should have a BMI of between 20 and 25. A person is considered obese if he or she has a BMI of 30 or higher.

Furthermore, obesity can be assessed even more easily by considering the waist to hip ratio. That means the more 'pear-shaped' you are, the

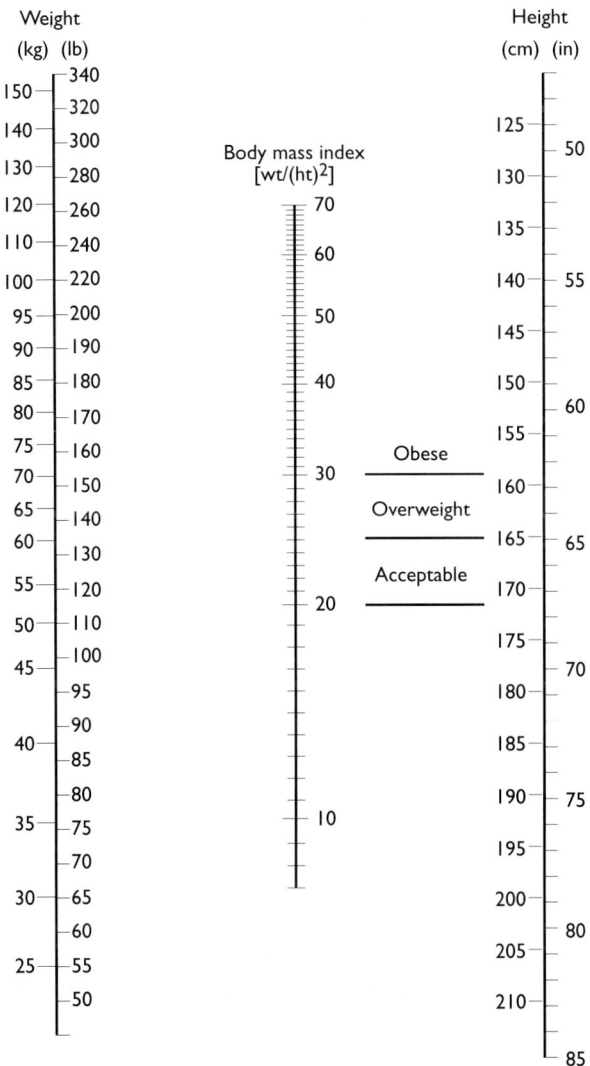

Figure 3.1 Chart (called a nomogram) for determining BMI. To use this nomogram, place a ruler or other straight edge between the body weight in pounds (without clothes) located on the left-hand column and the height in inches (without shoes) located on the right-hand column. The BMI is read from the middle of the scale.

more at risk you are. Your waist measurement should be less than your hip measurement. Easier still is just the waist measurement. Generally men with a waist over 40 inches (102 cm) in circumference are more at risk than those under 40 inches. Women with a waist measurement over 35 inches (89 cm) are at greater risk than those under 35 inches.

Oral contraceptives

Oral contraceptives or birth control pills alone are a low-level risk factor. However, if birth control pills are combined with certain other risk factors, such as smoking, or high blood pressure, then the risk of stroke increases dramatically. If you take the Pill you must not smoke and you must have regular health checks.

Physical inactivity

People who are physically inactive are more prone to have strokes.

Regular exercise will reduce your chance of having a stroke by 50%. Exercise lowers the blood pressure, slows the resting heart rate and reduces the stress on artery walls. Exercise also increases your general fitness and well-being.

Inactivity is not only a major risk factor for developing strokes and coronary artery disease, but it can also lead to high blood pressure, low levels of high-density lipoproteins (HDL or 'good cholesterol'), and diabetes. Exercising 30–40 minutes at least three or four times a week reduces blood pressure, raises HDL, and helps regulate insulin requirements. This level of exercise would be sufficient to reduce your chances of having a stroke.

Any type of physical exercise is beneficial, whether it be walking, running, swimming, playing sports, or gardening. The important thing is that you don't feel you are overdoing it. You should push yourself so you feel a little out of breath, but no more.

General health

Your general level of health will have an impact on your susceptibility to various diseases. It seems so obvious that everyone should try to maintain a healthy lifestyle, and to keep their body in good condition. The difficulty is that many of the things that people find enjoyable, such as smoking, eating fatty foods, and being physically inactive, are the very things that are so bad for you. As far as stroke is concerned, the following medical risks factors will increase the likelihood of having a stroke:

- High blood pressure (hypertension)
- High cholesterol level (hypercholesterolaemia)
- Hardening of the arteries (atherosclerosis)
- Carotid artery disease
- High red blood cell count
- Previous stroke/TIA
- Ischaemic heart disease (heart disease due to a narrowing of blood vessels within the heart).

These medical risk factors can be identified and treated by your GP and primary care team.

High blood pressure (hypertension)

High blood pressure is one of the most important risk factors for stroke and is a very common problem. It may affect one in four people and is more common as you get older. The chance of having a stroke in those with untreated high blood pressure (above 140/90; see below) is about seven times the risk of those with a normal or low blood pressure.

The number one cause of strokes is the failure to detect and control high blood pressure. Unfortunately, high blood pressure can have very few symptoms so regular checks are required. This is especially important for older people. If your blood pressure is normal at a check-up then you don't need it rechecked for 1–5 years. However, it may be necessary to recheck it more frequently if it is found to be elevated. Once treatment has returned the blood pressure to normal levels, then rechecks are required less frequently.

High blood pressure continually pounds the walls of blood vessels and can lead to strokes from bleeding from burst blood vessels and also from promoting the hardening of arteries and blood clots.

High blood pressure can be avoided and treatment can begin with a healthy diet low in animal fat and high in fruit and vegetables, avoiding adding salt to meals at meal times, avoiding excess alcohol intake, taking regular exercise, losing weight and avoiding smoking.

The blood pressure is given by two figures. The first higher reading represents the pressure exerted by the heart as it pumps the blood around the body after each contraction. This is called the *systolic* pressure. The second lower reading represents the resting pressure as the heart relaxes after the contraction. This is called the *diastolic* pressure. Many studies have been carried out on hundreds of thousands of people of all ages and backgrounds, and doctors have a very good indication of what normal blood pressure readings should be. The aim should be to keep one's blood pressure below 140/90.

High blood pressure is a risk factor for stroke whether either, or both, of the readings are raised. For example, an increased systolic (the first higher reading) blood pressure increases stroke risk by two to four times. Persistent blood pressure readings above 140/90 raise the risk of stroke by up to six times.

Your own doctor may prescribe medications to lower the blood pressure. It is such a common condition and treatment is so simple. You must take the tablets regularly according to the instructions. There are many different classes of tablets that can reduce blood pressure, and side effects, if they occur, can often be avoided by changing to a drug of a different class. Nowadays it is quite common to be on two, three, four or even more such drugs so as to limit the side effects of using high doses of individual drugs. A benefit is that the actions of different drugs are often complementary. Drug treatment should be accompanied by the lifestyle changes recommended above. Treatment of high blood pressure substantially reduces the risk of stroke by about 40%. Unfortunately, only about one-third of people who have high blood pressure have this controlled properly. At the very least, the blood pressure should be below 140/90. Blood pressure less than these readings is even better.

High blood pressure can be effectively controlled by a combination of regular exercise, a healthy diet, and medicines.

High cholesterol level (hypercholesterolaemia)

Cholesterol is an important chemical as it is used in the manufacture of steroid hormones, which are essential to the body's well-being. It is also a component of cell membranes. Everyone therefore has to have a certain amount of cholesterol in their body. However, as with many things, too much of a good thing can become a burden. There have been numerous medical studies that show that if the amount of cholesterol in the blood gets too high, then various unwelcome side effects occur, the main one being a hardening of the arteries due to the build-up of fatty deposits. This leads directly to high blood pressure and an increased risk of stroke (and other serious medical conditions as well).

Cholesterol is carried around in the blood attached to certain proteins. Most of it (about 70%) is attached to proteins called low density lipoproteins – LDL for short. The remainder is carried around attached to high density lipoproteins – HDL for short. The optimum values generally agreed by doctors are as follows:

- total cholesterol less than 5.2 (desirable);
- 5.2–6.5 (borderline);
- HDL cholesterol 0.8–1.8 (males), 0.8–2.3 (females);
- LDL cholesterol between 1.3 and 4.9.

In the large clinical trial known as the Heart Protection Study, patients with a total cholesterol level above 3.5 appeared to benefit from lipid-lowering therapy with a statin drug. In the light of this study, it may be necessary to treat stroke patients at a lower level of cholesterol than previously.

Hardening of the arteries (atherosclerosis)

Atherosclerosis is the process of gradually silting up the arteries in the body with time. It is often called 'hardening of the arteries'. It is encouraged by high blood pressure, smoking, high cholesterol levels, diabetes and by inflammatory states such as certain infections and rheumatoid arthritis.

Carotid artery disease

Fatty deposits found in the carotid artery (the main artery between the heart and brain) can block this important blood supply. Although there may be no symptoms, your doctor can often detect such a blockage by listening, with a stethoscope, to the sound of the blood pumping through the carotid artery. If an abnormal sound is heard (called a bruit, pronounced *bru-ee*), then a blockage is indicated. Depending on the amount of blockage, surgery (known as carotid endarterectomy) may be able to remove this build-up in the artery. For patients *without* symptoms due to a narrowing in the carotid arteries (i.e. an incidental finding), such operations are seldom offered in this country since the experts feel the risks outweigh the benefits, although often performed in European countries and in North America.

High red blood cell count
Although it is an uncommon cause of stroke, even a small increase in the red blood cell count can be a risk factor for stroke. This is because a high number of red blood cells will thicken the blood, which can lead to blood clots. Fortunately, the causes of this are often cigarette smoking and other lifestyle causes, so they can be easily corrected.

Previous stroke/TIA
The risk of a stroke increases greatly for a person who has already had a stroke. Unfortunately for those who have had a prior stroke, another stroke is 10 times more likely to occur than in those who have never had a stroke. This means that all risk factors that can be identified must be tackled. It also means secondary prevention therapy is vitally important.

Transient ischaemic attacks (TIAs)
TIAs are a warning sign of a possible future stroke. The risk is about 7.5% per year (1 in 13 patients will have a stroke after a TIA in the first year). Of those who have had one or more TIAs, more than a third will have a subsequent stroke. It is obviously essential to see a doctor right away if you or someone you know has any of the symptoms of a TIA or a stroke.

Other medical conditions
Diabetes
Diabetes leads to an increased risk of stroke. Although diabetes can be treated, people with the disease are still more likely to have a stroke. This is mainly because of the circulation problems that diabetes causes. If blood sugar remains high, brain damage at the time of a stroke may be more severe and widespread. This is not simply due to the higher

levels of glucose in the blood of diabetics. Diabetic patients more often have high blood pressure and high levels of cholesterol and other fats in the blood. All risk factors in diabetic patients must be treated. The incidence of stroke is greater for women who have diabetes than for men who have diabetes.

Obesity
Even being 10 kg (22 lbs) overweight will increase the risk of stroke. Obesity increases the chances of high blood pressure, heart problems, high cholesterol and diabetes. These are all risk factors for stroke as well.

Heart disease
Patients who have had a heart attack or who have angina are at higher risk of stroke. Normally those patients will have the risk factors for stroke attended to when they get treatment to help prevent their heart disease progressing.

Heart valve and rhythm disorders

Heart valve disease
The risk of stroke is increased when heart valve disease is present. This can be congenital (i.e. you are born with it) or damage to the heart by rheumatic heart disease. If this is discovered, you may be on medication to prevent strokes. The most important heart valve disease associated with the risk of stroke is mitral stenosis.

Atrial fibrillation (abnormal heart rhythm)
An irregular heart beat can be caused by atrial fibrillation. This heart rhythm disturbance is commoner as you get older and is associated with other heart and circulatory disorders. There is a chance that a clot can form in the fibrillating atrium due to blood standing still; if this clot moves to the brain it can cause a stroke.

Ischaemic heart disease, angina and heart attacks
Those who have signs of ischaemic heart disease, such as having had a heart attack, have an increased chance of sustaining a stroke. A clot

which can occur as a heart attack is healing may break off, causing an ischaemic stroke. This may occur in the hours or days after an acute myocardial infarction although modern treatment of heart attacks diminishes the risk of this serious complication.

Congestive heart failure
Patients with congestive heart failure are at increased risk of stroke.

Left ventricular hypertrophy
The word *hypertrophy* means enlargement due to overgrowth. Left ventricular hypertrophy (LVH) is a common consequence of high blood pressure and is due to over-strengthening or overgrowth of the main muscle of the heart, which is in the left ventricle (lower chamber) of the heart. This condition is associated with an increased chance of having a stroke.

If you have any of the above risk factors, then you need to be very careful about the things you can do something about. Controlling the three major risk factors for heart disease – cigarette/tobacco smoking, high blood cholesterol, and high blood pressure – can also reduce the risk of stroke.

Other factors

Socioeconomic factors

Studies have shown that stroke occurs at a lower age among those with lower incomes. The reasons for this are not completely understood. This may be partly due to the fact that other risk factors, e.g. smoking, may be commoner in these groups.

4 WHAT ARE THE SYMPTOMS OF A STROKE?

The structure of the brain

The brain consists of different parts as is illustrated in Figures 4.1–4.3.

The cerebral cortex consists of two halves. Because the nerves switch over after they leave the brain, the left side of the cortex controls movement and senses on the right side of the body so that a stroke in the left side will affect the right side of the body. Similarly, the right side of the cortex controls the movements and senses on the left side of the body, and a stroke in the left side will affect the right side of the body.

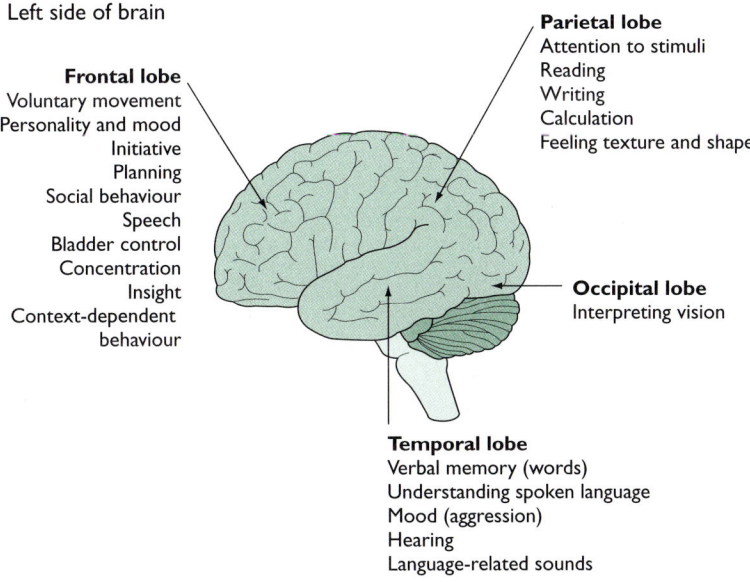

Figure 4.1 This shows all the complex things that the left half of the cerebral cortex does.

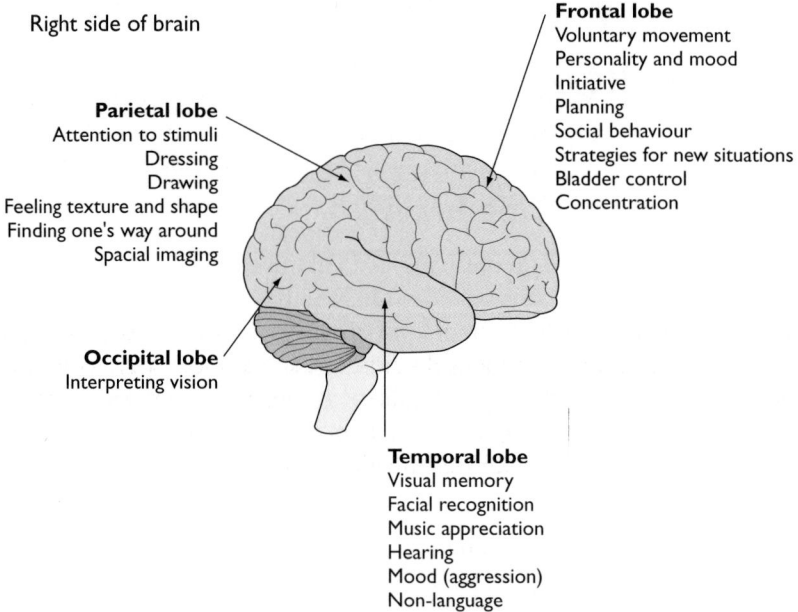

Figure 4.2 This shows all the complex things that the right half of the cerebral cortex does.

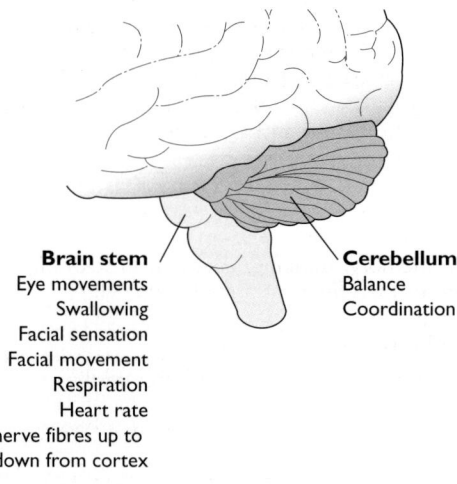

Figure 4.3 The brainstem and cerebellum.

Each half of the brain controls complex actions as illustrated in Figures 4.1 and 4.2.

There are other important parts of the brain including the brainstem and cerebellum (Figure 4.3). The brainstem is concerned with eye movements, swallowing, facial sensation and movement and all the fibres from the cortex pass through the brainstem. The cerebellum is concerned with balance and coordination.

Symptoms and signs

Doctors describe medical conditions in terms of *symptoms* and *signs*. *Symptoms* are what the patient describes to the doctor, such as loss of vision, tiredness, or difficulty in swallowing, whereas *signs* are what the doctor learns from carrying out an examination, such as fever or high blood pressure. This chapter deals with symptoms.

Table 4.1 Some effects of a stroke

1. Loss of consciousness
2. Weakness (hemiparesis) or paralysis (hemiplegia) on one side of the body that may affect the whole side or just the face, arm or leg. The weakness or paralysis is on the side of the body opposite the side of the brain affected by the stroke
3. Spasticity, stiffness in muscles, painful muscle spasms. This is a late effect of stroke and modern rehabilitation therapy is aimed to limit this
4. Problems with balance and/or coordination
5. Problems using language, including having difficulty understanding speech or writing (aphasia); and knowing the right words but having trouble saying them clearly (dysarthria)
6. Ignoring sensations on one side of the body or being unaware of them (bodily neglect or inattention)
7. Pain, numbness or odd sensations
8. Problems with memory, thinking, attention or learning
9. Being unaware of the effects of a stroke altogether
10. Difficulty swallowing (dysphagia)
11. Problems with bowel or bladder control
12. Fatigue (this symptom alone without other symptoms is rarely due to stroke)
13. Difficulty controlling emotions (emotional lability)
14. Depression and anxiety
15. Difficulties with daily tasks (due to a combination of effects above)

The possible symptoms of a stroke

These are shown in Table 4.1. Certain important symptoms are discussed further below.

Depending on the particular part of the brain affected, the following effects can occur after a stroke:

- Loss of consciousness. The majority of stroke patients do not lose consciousness
- Paralysis or weakness of one side of the body affecting the face, arm, or leg
- Loss of sensation affecting one side of the body
- Difficulty with speech and understanding
- Difficulty with swallowing and feeding
- Partial loss of vision to one side
- Memory loss or problems
- Loss of emotional control
- Fatigue
- Incontinence.

Difficulty with speech and understanding

Speech can be affected in different ways after a stroke.

Dysarthria

Dysarthria is a difficulty in making the sounds of speech, and is quite common even after a minor stroke. This is either because the muscles of the mouth and other muscles involved in voice production are weakened by the stroke or their coordinated movement is affected. Speech can be slurred and hard to understand because of this. Very rarely, it may be inaudible. However, the problem of dysarthria often responds well to exercises from a speech and language therapist.

Dysphasia

Dysphasia is a difficulty in the ability to communicate through speech but can also affect reading, writing, the use of simple communication cards and charts, and the ability to understand what is being said. It is due to damage to the part of the brain that controls language but only happens if these parts of the brain are affected by the stroke. The severity of this problem can vary greatly (and many people with a stroke are not affected at all). Some types of dysphasia produce differences in how well a person understands and some types affect what the speech sounds like. For many people with dysphasia it is frustrating to know what is going on around them but not be able to convey their worries and thoughts and not to understand explanations fully. Patients with dysphasia need extra time and patience but they do not need to be shouted at!

Speech and language therapists can accurately assess what the communication problem is and take time to explain to the patient, family and carers how this affects understanding and speaking. They will also arrange therapy to aid recovery. Often family and friends can be involved in this. Some people with dysphasia have mild communication problems and recover well and quickly, while others are left with a slowly recovering problem and sadly, some are left with a permanent communication difficulty.

Some communication equipment is available but very few patients are able to benefit from this.

Difficulty with swallowing and feeding

In the early phases after an acute stroke, it is quite common to have difficulty swallowing food and fluids. Choking is a common problem, as is difficulty chewing. Swallowing should be assessed soon after a stroke. As with other symptoms of a stroke, there can be minor or severe effects and recovery will take a variable time.

'No swallowing' or 'nil by mouth' instructions are often given until normal swallowing returns. Intravenous drips help replace fluids in hospital. Thickened fluids can be given to facilitate easier swallowing and as things improve normal fluids can be resumed. Solid foodstuffs can be given when recovery takes place and until then a specially staged diet with varying textures of foods can be used. Nasogastric feeding with a tube inserted up the back of the nose down to the stomach can facilitate feeding of liquid foodstuffs and fluids when swallowing is taking some time to recover. With persistent problems with swallowing, a PEG (percutaneous endoscopically placed gastrostomy) tube can be inserted through the abdominal wall into the stomach. The patient must, of course, be fit enough for this procedure.

Partial loss of vision to one side
Sight can be affected in several ways by a stroke or TIA, but generally involves some loss of vision in one eye.

Amaurosis fugax
This is a term used when the sight is temporarily lost in one eye due to an embolism originating in the carotid arteries (which connect the heart and the brain). An embolism is a blockage coming from somewhere else as opposed to a blockage occurring in the artery itself. The symptoms are often described as being like a curtain coming down over the eye. Fortunately, they only last minutes. If they lasted longer the blood supply to the eye would be interrupted for too long and blindness would result. This condition (a special type of TIA) needs prompt investigation.

Visual field defect
Visual field defects (quadrantanopia when one quadrant of vision is lost; hemianopia when half the visual field is lost), occur when a stroke affects either the visual cortex in the occipital pole of the brain, the part of the brain that interprets the images the eye sees, or the nerve pathway between the eyes and this area of the brain. Recovery can occur but many people have to learn to live with the defect. Unfortunately, it is not possible to continue holding a driving licence if the visual field defect is severe. Ophthalmology departments can arrange special visual field tests in uncertain cases.

Memory loss or problems
An acute stroke rarely causes memory loss on its own, although a severe stroke can affect many aspects of brain function. Memory loss can be a feature of 'multi-infarct dementia', which is due to recurrent strokes in specific areas of the brain associated with memory loss.

Loss of emotional control, mood changes, depression, frustration
After certain strokes, possibly due to changes in the neurotransmitter levels, emotional problems are sometimes seen. So-called 'emotionalism' may produce crying (or rarely) laughing with minimal or inappropriate stimuli.

Depressed mood, leading to clinical depression in some cases, will affect up to one-third of all hospitalized stroke patients. Anxiety is common after a stroke. Knowledge that there is improvement in most cases will help allay these fears. Special therapy with drugs (e.g. antidepressants) may help in selected cases. Other factors contributing to these changes will be previous psychiatric illness, boredom with the routine in the ward and lack of stimulation.

Fatigue

Fatigue after a stroke is a common symptom. This may be in part due to the healing process. Certainly taking part in a therapy regime to regain mobility will make a patient tired.

Incontinence, with loss of bladder control and bowel control

This seems to worry many patients, but is rarely seen except in the most severe cases. In-dwelling urinary catheters are used in those with coma or with severe mobility problems in the early phases but should be withdrawn when the patient recovers. Bowel problems are usually sorted out with regular toileting.

Warning signs

If you think you are having a stroke you must seek immediate medical attention. In certain circumstances, it is desirable to have drugs that will dissolve the blood clot (a process known as *thrombolysis*) that is causing a stroke. The time scale is very important as there are only 3–6 hours within which to administer this drug. Thrombolysis is used in the USA and Australia and some other countries. It is now licensed in Europe for use within 3 hours. It is vital this drug is given by expert personnel. It will only be available within certain centres.

Stroke is an attack on your brain. There is no time to waste. If someone is experiencing any of the following symptoms, treat them seriously and call for help:

- Sudden numbness or weakness in the face, arm or leg, especially if on one side of the body only.

- Sudden confusion, trouble speaking, trouble understanding.
- Sudden trouble seeing with one or both eyes.
- Sudden trouble walking; dizziness; loss of balance or coordination.
- Sudden severe headache with no known cause.

5 HOW IS A STROKE DIAGNOSED?

The majority of strokes occur suddenly and cause a weakness, numbness or problems with speech. The doctor will have taken a history of what happened to you and will perform a physical examination. A number of tests will then be organized.

The various possible symptoms of a stroke are described in Chapter 4. This chapter describes the various tests that can be carried out to enable the doctor to establish the *signs* of the condition, and eventually come up with a diagnosis.

Medical examination

The diagnosis of a stroke is a clinical diagnosis and no test can say a stroke has not occurred (e.g. rarely a CT scan will be normal even though the symptoms and signs of a stroke are present). A full clinical examination will be needed to make the diagnosis and many people feel they have never been examined in such detail before. The doctors will pay attention to pulse, blood pressure, listening to the heart, listening to the breathing, examining the abdomen as well as carefully examining the relevant parts of the body affected by the suspected stroke.

Blood tests

Routine blood tests will be carried out, and these are likely to include cholesterol, sugar and viscosity (the thickness or 'stickiness' of the blood) as well as full blood count (for anaemia) and urea and electrolytes (to check kidney function). There may also be other tests that the doctor wishes to carry out, especially if the patient is young.

Brain scans

Computerized tomography (CT) scan
This is a special type of x-ray scan of your head which is done to determine if a stroke has occurred or if the symptoms are due to any other problem. It is also able to determine whether the stroke is due to a bleed or a blockage. The doctors can also see where the damage has occurred and the size of the damaged area (Figures 5.1–5.5). The CT scan is therefore an extremely valuable diagnostic tool. It takes just over one minute to do once you are in the scanner.

Magnetic resonance imaging (MRI) scan
An MRI scan can be done as an alternative to a CT scan, but is not so readily available. It also takes longer to do than a CT scan. MRI scanners use powerful magnets (but no x-rays or other radiation) to detect the natural changes that occur in the body. Sometimes it is more detailed and precise than a CT scan (Figures 5.6–5.9).

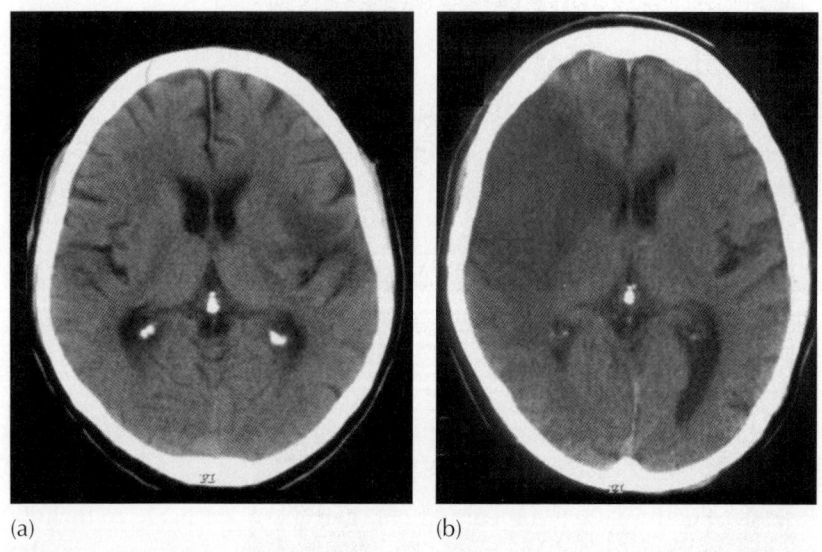

(a)   (b)

Figure 5.1 Cerebral infarction. (a) Part of the middle cerebral artery supply on the left is blocked. (b) Most, if not all, of the middle cerebral artery supply is blocked. The symptoms are more severe in those with more severe cerebral infarctions.

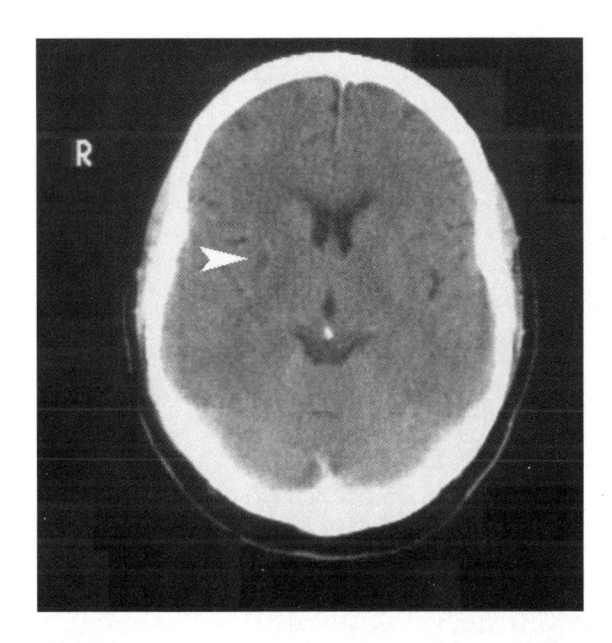

Figure 5.2 Smaller cerebral infarctions lead to fewer symptoms and can be difficult to detect (arrow). This patient had tingling and numbness down the left arm and leg which resolved after a few days.

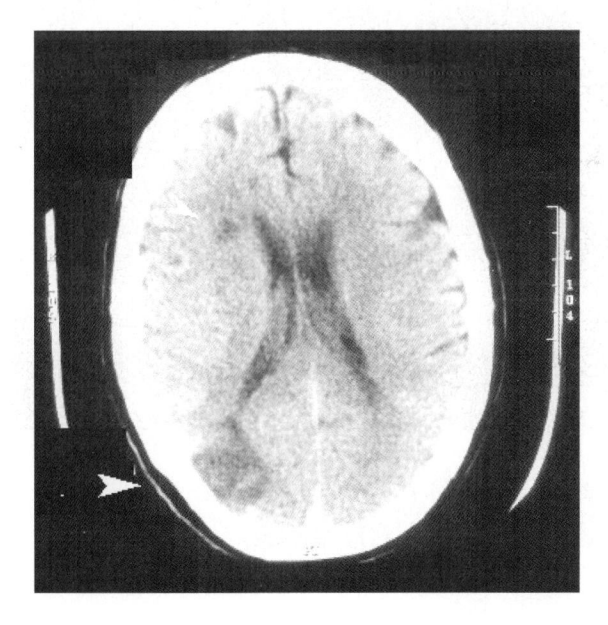

Figure 5.3 Sometimes multiple infarcts are seen on a CT scan.

29

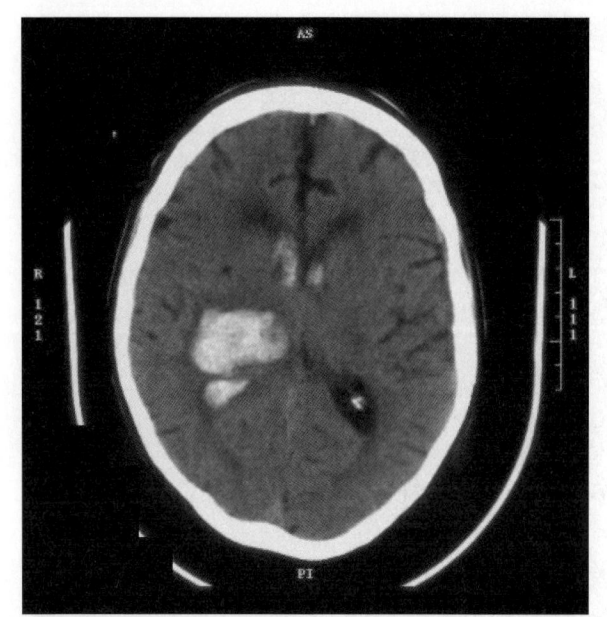

Figure 5.4 Cerebral haemorrhages are detected on CT scan. Deep haemorrhages (a) may be more serious than more superficial ones (b).

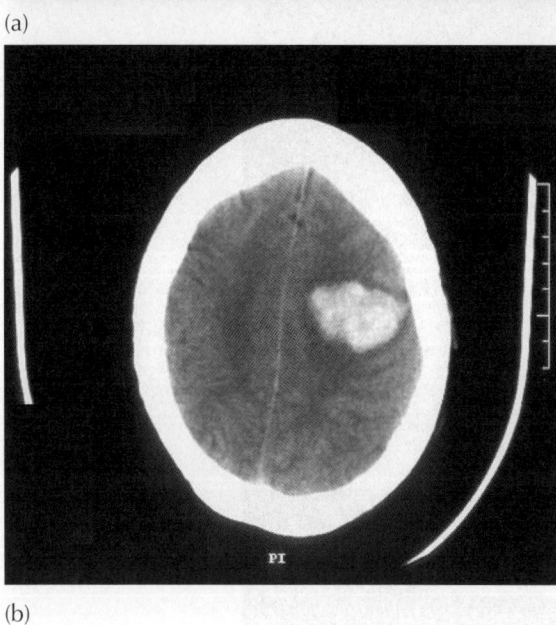

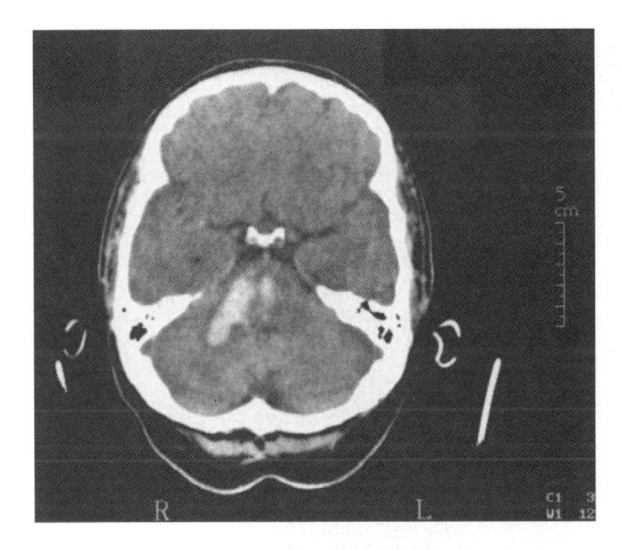

Figure 5.5 This CT scan shows a brainstem haemorrhage.

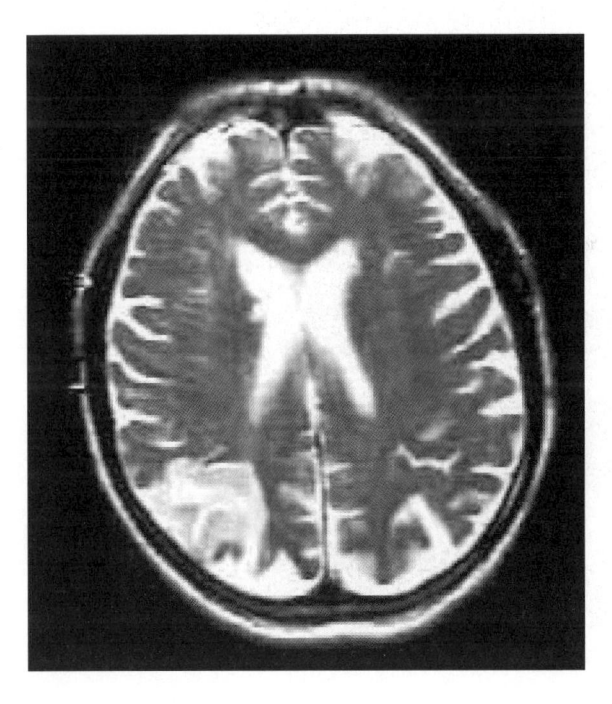

Figure 5.6 In this type of MRI scan the cerebral infarct shows up as a white area.

31

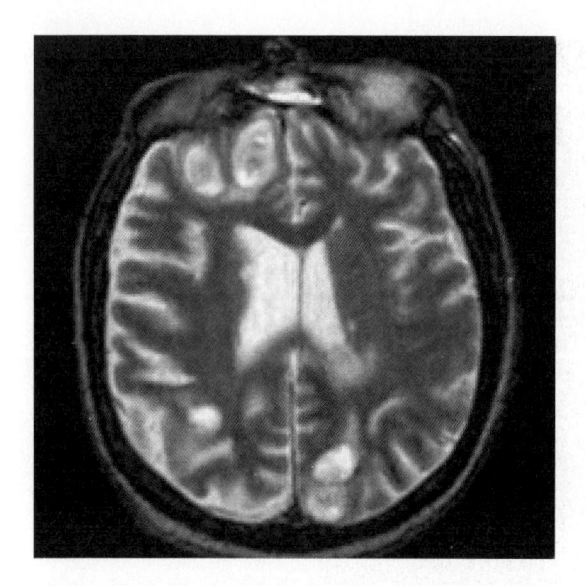

Figure 5.7 Multiple infarcts can sometimes be found, as in this patient with a cardiac source of embolism.

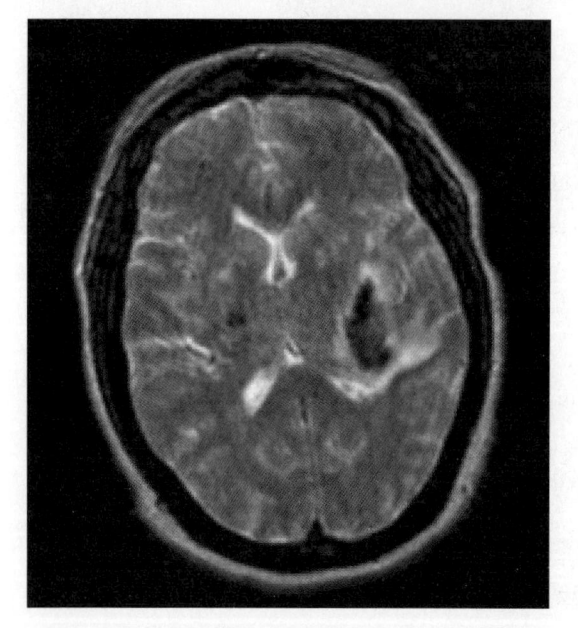

Figure 5.8 In this MRI scan the haemorrhage shows as a darker area in the brain due to different detection techniques used.

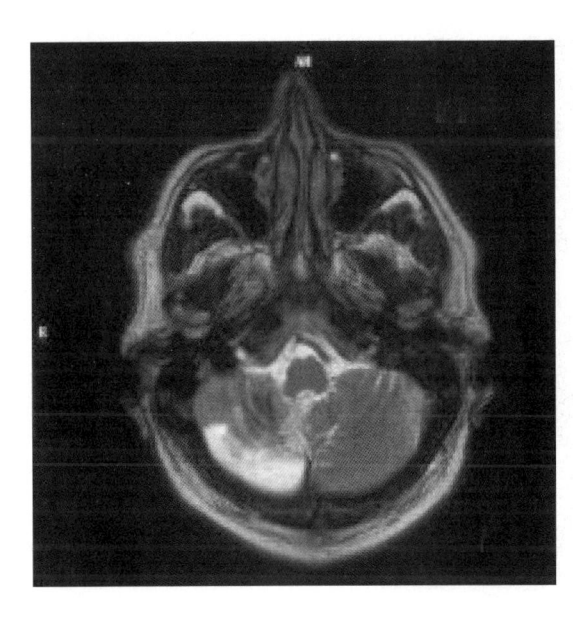

Figure 5.9 MRI scans are useful for investigating the cerebellum. This scan shows a cerebellar infarct (white area).

Other scans

Duplex Doppler of the carotid arteries

This is a special scan of the blood vessels (carotid arteries) on either side of your neck, which supply the brain with blood. It is done by using an ultrasound probe and is painless and harmless. The probe detects reflected ultrasound waves, which then generate a picture, just like the ultrasound that is used to look at unborn babies. Sometimes the carotid arteries have become furred up and narrowed and are causing a problem. If the narrowing is severe, your doctor may refer you to a vascular surgeon to discuss this more fully and see if they can operate to widen the artery. This is called a carotid endarterectomy.

Other tests

ECG (electrocardiogram)

An electrocardiograph machine has a number of electrical leads which are taped onto the chest in different positions. These then pick up the

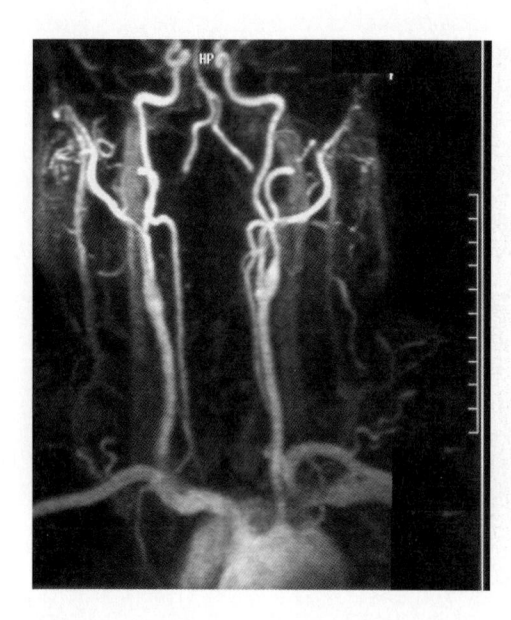

Figure 5.10 This MRA image shows normal arterial supply to the brain.

electrical activity of the heart and display it as a series of tracings, either on paper or on the screen of the machine. By looking at these tracings, the doctor can check the heart rate and rhythm and how it is functioning. It can also detect previous heart attacks, and damage caused by high blood pressure. Sometimes it is necessary to have a continuously monitored ECG over a 24-hour period, and this is done with a portable device carried around with you.

Echocardiogram

An echocardiogram is produced by a machine called an echocardiograph. This is an ultrasound type of device that measures the echoes of the ultrasound waves as they bounce back from the heart into the machine. This allows doctors to look at the structure of the heart while it is working. Strokes are sometimes caused by a broken piece of blood clot that has come from elsewhere. An echocardiogram may be done to see if the clot is likely to have come from the heart. Special treatment with anticoagulants would then be appropriate.

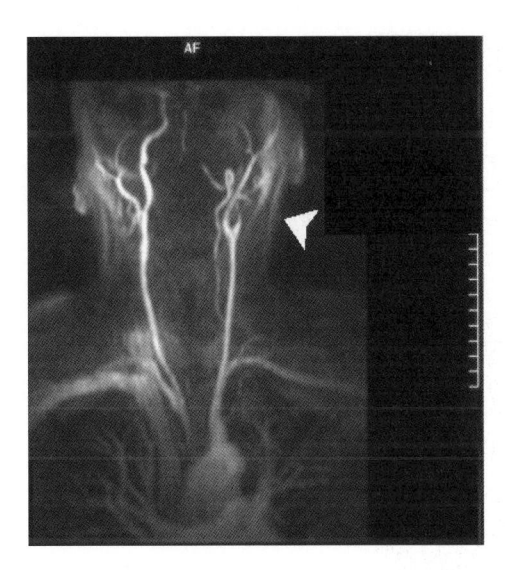

Figure 5.11 This MRA shows a blockage of the left internal carotid artery.

24-Hour blood pressure monitor
High blood pressure is one of the main causes of stroke and has to be carefully monitored after a stroke. The doctor may want to have a 24-hour continuous tracing of your blood pressure to have a better picture of when it is raised and this may affect how the doctor treats it. An automatic portable device will take blood pressure readings every 15–30 minutes for a 24-hour period. The 24-hour monitor is often called an ABPM (ambulatory blood pressure measurement).

Magnetic resonance angiography (MRA)
This is sometimes used to check for blockages in the carotid circulation, especially when it may be above the jaw (where it would not be accessible to duplex Doppler, see above) (Figures 5.10, 5.11).

Lumbar puncture
It may be necessary for the doctors in hospital to test the fluid that surrounds the brain (cerebrospinal fluid, CSF). This is done by performing

a lumbar puncture. A local anaesthetic is used and, contrary to common belief, is relatively painless.

Other tests (especially in younger patients)

Other tests may be necessary on various clotting factors and for certain genetic conditions associated with strokes at an early age. They are generally only appropriate for those younger than 40–45 years of age.

6 THE IDEAL CONSULTATION – WHAT SHOULD I TELL MY DOCTOR?

My symptoms

You must tell the doctor everything about what you feel and notice that is different.

- Is there a weakness – if so, where: face, arm, leg?
- Is there a loss of coordination or problems with balance – if so, where: face, arm, leg? Do you drop things or have difficulty, e.g. fastening things?
- Is there loss of sensation – if so, where: face, arm, leg?
- Is there a funny burning or pricking feeling – if so, where: face, arm, leg?
- Is your vision affected – if so, which visual field, or which eye?
- Is your speech slurred or is there a problem with the words coming out?
- Do you feel dizzy in addition to the other symptoms? Is this light-headedness or is the room spinning round?
- Do you have any other symptoms, e.g. headache – if so, where, and do you feel sick?

When they started

An accurate time line is essential.

- When were the first symptoms noticed?
- Did all the symptoms come on at once, or did they develop gradually over minutes or hours or days?
- When were they at their worst?
- Are they improving a little or a lot?

What you did about them

- Did you take any medication?
- Did it help or worsen the situation?
- Did you call anyone for help? If so, who?

Lifestyle

Information on lifestyle is important. If you are or were a smoker, information about when you started, when you stopped, and how much you smoked are all important details for the doctor to know. Alcohol intake is also important. Your occupation and hobbies should be revealed. What medication you are currently taking, both prescribed by your doctor, as well as any non-prescribed (over-the-counter) medicines, should be disclosed. Your past medical history may hold vital clues. You should be entirely open with your doctor regarding your personal habits since the consultation is entirely confidential.

Family history

This is very important. Are your parents alive or dead? What illnesses have they suffered from? What did they die from? How old were they when these things happened? Similar details will be needed about your siblings and your children. In some cases, aunts' and uncles' or cousins' information may be important. A family history of stroke, TIAs, heart attacks, angina, bypass grafts or angioplasties may be relevant as may a family history of high blood pressure, diabetes, or high cholesterol.

7 WHAT TREATMENTS ARE AVAILABLE?

There are basically three types of treatments available for stroke. These can be classified as *lifestyle treatments, medical treatments* and *surgical treatments*. In addition, physiotherapy, occupational therapy and speech therapy are invaluable aids.

Lifestyle treatments

Recovery from a stroke is usually due to teamwork, and you are an important member of the team, taking an active part in your own health.

It is important to minimize the risk of having a further stroke. Some risk factors cannot be changed, for instance your age, gender and family history. Other risk factors can be treated by drugs and surgery, and there are some which as well as being treated in this way can also be changed by the way you live your life. These are called modifiable risk or *lifestyle* factors and are changes you need to incorporate into your lifestyle. This is something positive that you can do.

High blood pressure

This is linked with strokes and heart attacks. Find out what your blood pressure is and if it needs to be reduced. Ways of reducing your blood pressure have already been mentioned (see page 13), but include losing weight, taking regular exercise, and avoiding salt. Your doctor may recommend taking tablets if the above measures are not effective on their own.

Watching your diet

There are a number of changes that can be made to your diet, which will be beneficial. Eating more fruit and vegetables is certainly beneficial. Reducing animal fats (butter, cheese, cream, fatty meat) and refined carbohydrates (sugar, biscuits, cakes) is useful. Consuming more fibre is beneficial. It has been suggested that eating one to two servings more of fruit and vegetables per day can reduce stroke risk by about 40%.

Diet checklist
- Increase fibre
- Reduce fat intake
- Reduce salt intake
- Aim to eat 5 portions or more of fruit and vegetables daily.

Weight

Being overweight contributes not only to high blood pressure, but also has been associated with higher levels of fat and blood glucose. Try to reduce the overall amount of food that you eat and increase physical activity. Think about your day and how you could increase the physical activity within it or join an exercise class. This does not have to mean going to the local gym to do aerobics; see if there is a gentle exercise programme in your area. There are some groups around called 'Extend' that do exercises sitting on a chair; alternatively, you could try doing some at home. Even if you have a 'bad side', you can still exercise the good one, so try to do as much as you can within your limitations. An increase in physical activity can produce a protective effect by lowering blood pressure, reducing fat and sugar levels in the body and generally making you feel better.

Salt intake

We need to have some salt in our diet, but too much can increase blood pressure. Our bodies need the sodium from salt but it is estimated that we only need about three-quarters of a teaspoon a day. Try not to add salt when cooking or at the table when eating. It is found naturally in many foods, and processed foods can often have high amounts of salt in them. Have a look at the ingredients label to see what the content is. There are a number of items produced that have not had extra salt added, so look for the no-added-salt or reduced-salt varieties at the supermarket.

Fats

The body has good and bad fats and the levels of these as well as their ratio to each other is important. The main fat in the bloodstream is cholesterol. We need cholesterol and it is produced naturally by the body as well as from the food we eat. Some people produce more than is needed and the problem can run in families. It is important to keep the levels of fats in the blood within the normal limits given by the doctor (see page 15) as fat can be deposited on to the walls of the blood vessels, furring them up and causing a narrowing or blocking them. There are many ways of reducing your fat intake: never fry, trim fatty meat, switch to skimmed or semi-skimmed milk and use a low fat spread. When cooking, skim fat off the top of dishes as it rises. Look at the fat content of foods. There are lots of low-fat alternatives around now. Check the type of fat, and use poly- and monounsaturated fats if possible. Limit the amount of eggs you eat in a week, as the yolks are very high in cholesterol, and cut down on the amount of cheese eaten. Try low-fat varieties or some of the soft cheeses such as Brie that have less fat in them. There are also some foods that claim to lower cholesterol levels but these can be expensive. Try to change other aspects of your diet to compensate for the reduction in fat. Eat more fruit and vegetables. The recommendations are 5 portions a day – a glass of fruit juice counts as one. Fruit and vegetables contain lots of vitamins and eating more of them will increase your intake of fibre. Increase the amount of carbohydrate (rice, pasta and bread, for example) in your diet for some more energy.

Diet dos and don'ts

Do:

- eat fruit and vegetables – at least five servings a day;
- go for skimmed milk and low-fat yoghurts and cheese, e.g. cottage cheese;
- base your diet around starchy foods like potatoes, whole grains like rice, barley, couscous, pasta, yam, sweet potatoes – eat some in every meal;
- choose low-fat meat and poultry like chicken, turkey, rabbit and game. Oily fish is a good source of protein as it contains omega-3 fats which help protect blood vessels;

- save fatty, sugary foods for occasional treats.

Don't:

- fry – grilling, steaming, baking or microwaving are healthier than frying;
- consume too many fats – especially saturated fats and transfatty acids found in some margarines;
- eat too many processed foods and snacks which are usually high in salt (as well as sugar and often saturated fat).

Alcohol

Too much alcohol may raise your blood pressure, therefore increasing the risk of stroke. Although UK government guidelines as to safe levels are now 28 units a week for men, and 21 units a week for women, many health education groups still recommend 21 units for men and 14 units for women. A unit is approximately one glass of wine, one measure of spirits, or one half pint of beer. Just as important is the way you drink. It is better for instance to have a glass of wine every night, than 7 glasses on a Saturday night!

Diabetes

People who have diabetes are at a higher risk of stroke. Although you can't alter the fact that you have diabetes, you can ensure that you keep it well controlled by watching the sugar intake in your diet, taking regular blood glucose measurements, and taking medications if instructed. Your own doctor will give you advice.

There are some other factors in your lifestyle that you can do something about.

Stress

Stress itself is not a proven cause of stroke, but there is a relationship between stress and high blood pressure. It can be difficult to reduce stress levels within your life but try to address them, and make positive steps towards relaxation. Meditation or yoga can help and tapes for relaxation are available.

Smoking

If you smoke, giving it up is the most important thing you could do. The risk of a further stroke gets less immediately you give up and within 5 years your risk of stroke will be the same as a non-smoker. Smoking makes the blood thicker and more likely to clot, it damages the blood vessels by making them less elastic, and can narrow them, causing blockages. It also has a bad effect on cholesterol levels. Smoking also causes heart attacks, lung cancer and bronchitis and costs a lot of money. There is help available. It is well recognized that it can be very difficult to give up and many health centres and hospitals run smoking cessation clinics. There is a Smoking Helpline and there are now a number of replacement therapies available through prescription to help you.

Handy tips to stop smoking

Set yourself a date to stop in the future and keep a diary of when you smoke. This will highlight the most important times you smoke and help you to change your routine at these times to overcome the desire for a cigarette. See if a friend will stop with you. Get rid of all cigarettes and lighters from the house and ask people not to smoke in the house. Remember, if you fail, try again, as some people don't manage it at the first attempt.

Medical treatments

Drugs

Treatment with drugs is designed to treat the effects of stroke, to prevent complications and to help treat risk factors in the hope of preventing a further stroke occurring. There are many drugs that can be used. They may include the following (see also Chapter 8, page 53):

- Thrombolytic (clot dissolving) drugs may help improve outcome after an ischaemic stroke. Unfortunately they have to be given very soon after the onset of a stroke and not many people arrive at hospital within the time limits. Also, many patients are not suitable for this therapy for many reasons This therapy may not be available at your local hospital.

- Trials are also under way on drugs designed to limit the extent of damage to the brain tissue. None has yet proven effective in humans but the search is still on.
- Antiplatelet drugs that make the blood less sticky and help reduce its tendency to clot, such as aspirin, dipyridamole and clopidogrel. Early use of aspirin in ischaemic stroke will be beneficial.
- Anticoagulant drugs (such as warfarin) that reduce clotting factors in the blood so it is less likely to clot in atrial fibrillation and when an ischaemic stroke occurs as a complication of a heart attack.
- Cholesterol-lowering drugs to treat atherosclerosis.
- Antihypertensive drugs which lower the blood pressure.
- Paracetamol to limit the extent of fever.
- Antibiotics to treat infections.

Surgical treatment

There are a number of operations which may be of help to certain patients under certain circumstances. These are specialist procedures, however, which would be performed by either a neurosurgeon or a vascular surgeon, and are definitely not suitable for everyone.

Carotid endarterectomy

This is an operation which removes the blockage of fatty material from inside the carotid artery on the affected side of the brain, but not when the blockage is actually inside the skull. It is only advised if the blockage is severe. This operation is not suitable for everyone – some people are too frail or there may be other reasons not to operate. It certainly cannot be done when the artery is completely blocked. Timing is also important – 6 months after the stroke the risks of surgery probably outweigh any benefit. Individual cases need to be carefully evaluated by the vascular surgeon.

Carotid angioplasty

An alternative to carotid endarterectomy is to open up the blocked arteries with a balloon, an operation known as carotid angioplasty. This is done under x-ray guidance, but it is also a specialist procedure only performed in certain hospitals. Like carotid endarterectomy, it is impossible to do when the artery is completely blocked.

Surgery within the skull

Any arteries that are blocked inside the skull cannot be treated surgically. However, it is possible in some situations to remove the blood that has escaped during a haemorrhagic stroke, caused by a burst blood vessel. This is a very specialist procedure that would only be performed by experienced neurosurgeons. It is important to say that this would not benefit everyone. Patients who have had really bad bleeds would be extremely unlikely to improve and may actually get worse after such a procedure. Guidance from your specialist is essential.

Physiotherapy, occupational therapy and speech therapy

Rehabilitation

Treatment of stroke patients in a dedicated stroke unit is known to achieve a better outcome for stroke patients. Part of the reason for this, apart from appropriate use of diagnostic and treatment facilities, is because the patient has access to a multidisciplinary team. This includes doctors and nurses and rehabilitation therapists – physiotherapists (or physical therapists), occupational therapists and speech and language therapists. Although between two and four out of ten people who have had strokes are currently treated at home, this is only appropriate for a few patients. Research has shown conclusively that organized stroke care in a dedicated stroke unit saves lives and reduces disability. Of those people who survive a stroke, around half will be left with some significant disability. All the same, the brain is remarkably adaptable and in the months or years after a stroke many cells that have sustained damage recover some of their function. At the same time, other areas of the brain take over the functions performed by the cells that have died. The time it takes to recover is extremely variable. However, commonly people have a surge of recovery in the weeks following a stroke followed by a slower recovery over the next year to 18 months or so. The aim of rehabilitation is to encourage and enhance this process. It may include:

- help to aid physical recovery;
- help in managing the physical, emotional and social effects of stroke;
- aids and encouragement to allow patients to become as independent as possible;
- medical and other help to prevent potential medical or psychological complications.

The process of rehabilitation

Rehabilitation is a complex process and may include physiotherapy, occupational therapy and speech and language therapy. It will be tailored to the individual's needs, and assessments made at the initial period after the stroke will be reviewed in the light of recovery. Other disciplines such as social workers, dieticians and chiropodists can be 'drafted in' to help in the rehabilitation process. A great deal of work is currently going on to discover the best and most appropriate kind of rehabilitation and how long it should last.

The success of rehabilitation depends on:

- amount of damage that the brain has suffered;
- skill on the part of the rehabilitation team;
- cooperation of family and friends. Caring family/friends can be one of the most important factors in rehabilitation;
- timing of rehabilitation – the earlier it begins the more likely survivors are to regain lost abilities and skills.

After a period of in-patient rehabilitation, the programme can be continued at home with rehabilitation teams operating in the community, or by regular visits to out-patients or day hospital. The majority of stroke patients make a significant recovery and can be discharged from the initial programme of rehabilitation.

Support at home

A number of useful agencies can help patients with disabilities to cope at home. They are often coordinated by local Social Work departments. Home helps and Meals on Wheels can help. District nursing services are also immensely useful.

8 RECOVERY AND COMPLICATIONS

What are the chances of recovery?

The chances of recovery are actually very high and most patients do make progress. However, there is no doubt that stroke can be a very serious disease. The outlook or prognosis is largely dependent on factors such as how much of the brain has been damaged. The more damage there is, the lower the chance of a full recovery. As a consequence, there is a higher chance of dying early after the stroke when the stroke is severe.

Of the patients admitted to hospital with a stroke, about one-quarter will get a bit worse after admission (before showing signs of improvement). About one in twelve to one in five of patients admitted to hospital may die because their stroke is so severe. By one year after a stroke up to one-quarter of patients may have died and by 5 years about one-half will have died. Survival will be improved if the stroke is mild and secondary prevention treatment is used. In the first year after a stroke about one in twelve patients may have a recurrent event and by 5 years more than a quarter will have a further stroke. Modern treatment tends to reduce the chances of this happening.

What complications can occur?

Infections

Chest infections

Chest infections can be a problem after a stroke, especially when swallowing is affected. Saliva and food or drink can get into the lungs and lodge there. Difficulty in coughing due to lack of a cough reflex and to muscle paralysis can prevent this material from being cleared properly, and infections can easily start. Lying flat after a stroke is another potential hazard. It may be necessary to monitor the amount of oxygen in the blood, and to give oxygen if necessary. Antibiotics may also be needed.

Urinary infections

Urinary tract infections are common after a stroke. The use of a urinary catheter, even temporarily, can increase the risk of this occurring. Hygiene problems associated with incontinence in those with very severe strokes is a contributory factor. Treatment with antibiotics may be necessary.

Skin problems

Skin ulceration due to pressure sores can be avoided by careful nursing. Wet skin due to incontinence, poor circulation, lack of sensation in a paralysed limb, undernourishment and obesity are some of the factors which can make these problems more liable to happen.

Blood clots

Blood clots deep within the veins are a risk after stroke and can prove fatal. A difficulty is that they are not always readily apparent to the doctor or nurse. These clots usually start in a paralysed leg or in the pelvis. Clots in the leg can cause swelling, heat and redness over the affected part, and may therefore be detectable due to these symptoms. The risk is that they may break off and travel to the lung, causing a *pulmonary thromboembolism* (a blood clot in the lung). This can have either no symptoms, or it can cause chest pain, or the coughing up of blood. In rare cases, it can lead to sudden death. Avoidance strategies include early mobilization and wearing special compression stockings that are designed to minimize the risk of clot formation. Drugs that prevent the blood from clotting, such as aspirin, may also be of benefit and, under specialist supervision, heparin and similar medications.

Joint problems

Joint problems are rare after a stroke unless the patient is already suffering from a joint disease such as rheumatoid arthritis or osteoarthritis. However, any joint can become painful if it is positioned poorly. Most physiotherapists, occupational therapists and nurses are skilled in the proper positioning of stroke patients so that these potential problems are avoided.

Shoulder joint pain in the affected arm is quite common after a stroke. One of the causes is stretching of the joint capsule of the affected shoulder joint and care should be taken to minimize this. Unfortunately, if there is lack of normal sensation in the affected side, the patient may be unaware that their arm is pulling that shoulder out of place.

Simple pain killers such as paracetamol may help, but non-steroidal anti-inflammatory drugs, such as ibuprofen, and the stronger morphine-related drugs may be needed.

Seizures

Epileptic seizures are an unusual complication of stroke but a frightening one if they do occur. If they occur in the first few days after the stroke, they are likely to be due to the immediate effects of the stroke itself, while if they occur later they are probably due to scar tissue that has formed after the stroke. Many doctors would accept that one or more seizures due to a stroke should be treated with anticonvulsant drugs. However, this would depend on the severity of the seizure, the presence of other illnesses, whether and which other drugs are being taken, and whether the person was on their own for long periods. Naturally, epileptic seizures will affect the fitness to drive and must be reported to the DVLA (Driver and Vehicle Licensing Agency).

Constipation

Bowel function can slow down after a stroke and lead to constipation. Eating regular meals which contain roughage, such as wholemeal bread and vegetables, should be encouraged. It is also important to drink plenty of fluids and to keep as active as possible.

Mood disorders

Depression is common after a stroke, and talking to others can be a great help. There is help available and there is no shame in asking for it. Treatment with an antidepressant drug may help.

After a stroke some people become emotionally labile – this means they may burst out laughing or crying at unexpected moments. This should improve over time but it may also affect them to such an extent that it hampers recovery. The doctor may be able to prescribe some medication to help.

Anxiety is especially common. Worrying about what the future holds is seldom helpful. Fortunately, as things improve after the stroke, then anxiety levels improve too.

Falls and fractures

Falls are common, especially in the early recovery phase after a stroke. They can reduce confidence and cause painful bruising but often are minor. They can be due to muscle weakness or a lack of coordination, or to just being overambitious. Sensible attention to exercise regimens and relying on help of others often avoids falls. In hospitals, the use of special hoists and equipment often minimizes falls as well as reducing damage to nurses' and physiotherapists' backs! Some falls are often to be expected in a rehabilitation programme after a stroke and often the physiotherapist will give advice on how to rise after a fall.

Fractures are not common after a stroke, although a fall in a patient with osteoporosis can result in a fractured wrist or hip. Exercising as much as possible after a stroke is thought to be beneficial in slowing the development of osteoporosis.

Prevention of further strokes

Lifestyle treatments

There are various changes in your lifestyle that will help you feel fitter and healthier and help reduce your risk of stroke. They include:

Stop smoking
Stop smoking if necessary. Even if you've tried to quit before, it's worth trying again. Stop smoking aids like nicotine patches, complementary therapies such as acupuncture and joining a stop smoking group can often help motivation.

Alcohol

Stick to safe alcohol limits: that's 14 units a week for women and 21 for men. A unit = half a pint of beer, a glass of wine, or a single pub measure of spirits.

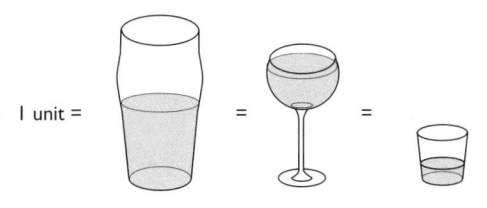

I unit = [pint glass] = [wine glass] = [tumbler]

Avoid binge drinking: i.e. drinking a lot of alcoholic drinks in a short space of time.

Weight

Watch your weight: being overweight stresses the heart and increases the risk of high blood pressure. Your doctor can tell you what's healthy for you. The best way to lose weight is a low-fat diet and regular activity. You may find it motivating to join a slimming club.

Exercise

Regular physical activity can help improve the condition of the heart, enhance the circulation, lower blood pressure, lower cholesterol levels and help keep weight down, so helping reduce the risk of stroke. It can also help you feel more energetic and cheerful. The gym need not be the only way to exercise. Walking to the shops, using the stairs instead of the lift, getting off the bus a stop earlier, and going for a longer brisk walk at weekends can all improve aerobic capacity. Improving the anaerobic capacity by increasing the heart rate can be very helpful. Other activities for the more adventurous are to be encouraged and include tennis, dance classes, cycling, or swimming. If your stroke has affected your mobility, the doctor or physiotherapist can help devise a suitable activity plan. Always check with your doctor before starting an exercise programme and do not overdo it! It would be best to aim to do some exercise each day and at least 30 minutes on 5 days out of 7. Even walking 20 minutes a day will reduce the risk of stroke.

Exercise dos and don'ts

Do:
- check with your doctor before starting to exercise.
- choose an activity you enjoy – you're more likely to keep it up.
- try to do 30 minutes of moderate exercise 5 days a week.
- aim to do some form of aerobic exercise every day.
- choose exercise suitable to your level – your doctor, physiotherapist or fitness trainer at the gym can advise.
- *remember* – just 20 minutes walking a day reduces the risk of stroke.

Don't:
- overdo it – small regular amounts are best. Avoid very vigorous activity.
- continue exercising if you feel pain, dizzy, sick or tired.
- exercise if you feel unwell or have an infection.
- do weight-lifting or other isometric exercise (in which you use resistance) – they can increase blood pressure.

Stay calm

Stress may be linked to high blood pressure. Learning stress management techniques and making time for rest and relaxation can only be good for you. This needn't be passive: practices such as yoga or meditation can help.

Share your feelings

Bottling up your feelings can often make worries appear larger than they are. Sharing feelings and worries can help ease the burden.

Take control

An event such as a stroke can be very shocking and depressing. However, taking control of your life by doing as much as you can to reduce your risk can be a very positive step and help to banish feelings of depression.

Get support

There's a whole range of statutory and voluntary support services out there for people who have had strokes (see Appendix).

Medication
Drugs such as antiplatelet medicines (e.g. aspirin and others) may be recommended to prevent stroke in those thought to be at risk. See below.

Medical treatments

Aspirin
Aspirin is taken to prevent platelets (small structures in blood involved in clotting) sticking together too readily. Many people regard it as 'thinning the blood' but no drug actually does this. Aspirin prevents the platelets clumping together.

Dipyridamole MR (modified release)
Dipyridamole MR (Persantin Retard) also prevents platelets sticking together too readily. There are many people who take a combination of aspirin and Persantin Retard, which may be superior to aspirin alone in preventing further events. The modified-release preparation of Persantin is the one that has been proven effective. This is available on its own to use with your own aspirin or a combination product with aspirin in it (Asasantin Retard).

Clopidogrel
Clopidogrel is another powerful drug that prevents platelets sticking together. It may be more powerful than aspirin and can also be used in those who cannot tolerate aspirin.

Warfarin
Warfarin is an anticoagulant and stops the blood clotting by a different mechanism from the antiplatelet drugs above. You may be on this if you suffer from atrial fibrillation (fluttering of the heart). The dose of warfarin has to be carefully monitored: this is done by regular special blood testing to see how prolonged the blood clotting is. Warfarin is not suitable for everyone with atrial fibrillation. There are other reasons for taking warfarin and your GP will supervise carefully.

Statin drugs
Statin drugs, such as simvastatin, pravastatin, fluvastatin and atorvastatin, are used to lower the cholesterol, and they may have other

beneficial effects on the blood vessels themselves as well as slowing down the progression of fatty deposits.

Blood pressure lowering drugs
Blood pressure lowering tablets such as ACE inhibitors (e.g. perindopril and ramipril) and diuretics (indapamide, bendrofluazide, etc.) can be used after a stroke. Some can even be used in those people with normal blood pressures to reduce the risk of further stroke. There are many different types of blood pressure lowering tablets and you may need to be on several different types to gain maximum effect.

Diabetes
It is important to have good blood glucose control. Diet, oral hypoglycaemic drugs and/or insulin regimens may be necessary. Other risk factors including stopping smoking, treating hypertension and treating abnormal blood lipids are very important.

Note
Never start or stop medication without consulting your doctor.

9 FREQUENTLY ASKED QUESTIONS

Why me?

Strokes happen for many different reasons and are usually sudden. This can cause upset and shock to the patient and the family. There is no definite reason 'why me' – we can only help to identify causes that may have contributed to the stroke and minimize the risk of it happening again.

Why am I so tired?

This is very common and is because the body is recovering from the stroke. It takes more effort and concentration to do the smallest of things that would have been taken for granted before. Learning to pace oneself and taking rests when feeling tired will help.

When will I recover?

Most people recover well and fully after an acute stroke. It may take some time and sometimes the recovery is not quite as full as might be hoped, but the majority will be well enough to manage independently. If help is required, there are numerous gadgets and aids that can help around the house. Lots of agencies can help. Sadly, however, some people never recover completely from their stroke, but at least they will be better than they were immediately after it happened. Recovery can actually continue for a number of years, albeit at a slow rate. Much will depend on the severity of the stroke and no two patients are identical. A positive attitude to your recovery will help.

Can I exercise?

Regular activity will help lower the blood pressure and cholesterol and help control weight. However, a doctor's advice should be sought before exercising. Gentle activity such as swimming is ideal. If active exercise is not possible, something like tai chi could prove beneficial.

Why is my memory not so good?

Minor memory problems after stroke are very common, but the degree to which people are affected can vary dramatically. Many people find their short-term memory is affected and that it is harder to remember new information, and that recalling information also takes longer. Concentration can be affected too. Very rarely does a stroke lead to a dementing illness and medications that are used to prevent further strokes will generally be useful in preventing some types of dementia.

When can I start driving again?

The DVLA has strict guidelines about who may or may not drive a car. Anyone who has had a stroke or a TIA should refrain from driving for a month after recovery. You may resume driving after this time if recovery is satisfactory. You don't have to notify the DVLA unless there is residual neurological deficit. They are especially concerned about visual field defects, cognitive defects and impaired limb function – minor weaknesses alone will not require notification

Special rules apply to Group 2 users (lorries, buses, minibuses etc.). Twelve month suspension of licence is usual and re-licence will depend on satisfactory medical reports.

If you have had a neurosurgical operation there are 6 to 12 months off driving, and epilepsy will mean a longer break (see DVLA website).

If you have frequent TIAs, you should not drive until you have had a 3-month period free from attacks. You should see your own doctor before starting to drive again to ensure that you are fit enough and he will give you further advice. You may have to inform the DVLA and have further assessment. It is possible to have adaptations made to your car to help with driving and there are mobility centres that can offer advice and help. Your insurance company must be informed both about your stroke or TIA and also if any modifications have been made to your car.

Remember: giving up driving until you are safe to drive again makes sense to you, your loved ones and to other road users.

The DVLA have to be notified if, after this month has passed, you are still not well enough to drive.

If you or your doctor would like further clarification or are unsure whether notification is required, advice can be obtained from the Drivers Medical Unit, DVLA, Longview Road, Swansea, SA6 7JL, Tel: 0870 6000 301, www.dvla.gov.uk. Once the DVLA has been notified, they will send you a questionnaire to fill in and ask your permission to contact your doctor for further information about your condition if necessary.

Is it safe to have sex?

Relationships are very important and regaining an active sex life after a stroke should be encouraged. It can be difficult for a number of reasons, however. There can be a number of different aspects to this, which may be the cause of problems after a stroke: the emotional, physical and the psychological as well as the effects of some medications. It is not dangerous to have sex; whilst it will raise the blood pressure it will not raise it to levels that will cause a stroke. The best way to deal with any problems is to talk and share feelings, not only with your partner, but you may also find your doctor or nurse able to help or counselling may help if you find that difficult. Two of the associations that may be able to help are Discern and SPOD (see Appendix).

Can I go on holiday?

The answer is yes. Holidays are good for you once you have recovered. Flying is no problem – if you have mobility difficulties do let the airline known in advance – they will be able to help.

If you have had a very recent stroke or a DVT (deep vein thrombosis) in the past or if you have paralysis remaining in the lower limbs, you may be at a higher risk of a DVT if you are on a long flight. To avoid this, wear comfortable shoes, drink plenty of water, use support stockings. Some people believe low-dose aspirin or injections of anticoagulant (low molecular weight heparin) may help, but there is no evidence to back this up. Your own doctor can give you individual advice if necessary.

10 CASE STUDIES

These case studies are an amalgamation of real situations and illustrate certain aspects of the diagnosis and treatment. Every patient presents individual problems that require individual solutions. There is no such thing as a 'standard' stroke patient.

Case 1

Mrs A is a 54-year-old who awoke one morning to find her right side was weak and had a loss of sensation. Her arm had virtually no movement, there was only a mild weakness in her leg and her face was drooped, causing slurred speech. Mrs A lives with her husband and they realized that she had had a stroke and dialled 999.

She was admitted to hospital where the doctors obtained a history of the event and the past medical history.

Mrs A had a number of risk factors for having a stroke:

- She was diabetic, controlled by diet.
- She had hypertension controlled by atenolol, bendrofluazide and ramipril.
- Previous event: a transient ischaemic attack 6 weeks earlier. Her right arm had been transiently weak for 10 minutes.
- Family history: her father died of a stroke at the age of 67.

Her other medications were:

- Prempak-C (HRT)
- aspirin, which had been started after the TIA
- ranitidine (she had been experiencing some oesophageal reflux problems).

On admission the doctors examined her and it appeared that she had also some mild word-finding problems and the tone of her muscles was increased in her arm and leg. Power was reduced in the right side of the face, arm and leg.

Routine tests

- Blood pressure was 187/89, pulse 80 and regular. Temperature was normal.
- ECG was normal.
- CT scan showed an infarct in the left middle cerebral artery territory.
- A carotid Doppler scan of the neck vessels was normal.
- Blood tests were within normal limits apart from the cholesterol which was raised at 6.1 mmol/l.

To see if she had any problems with swallowing, which can be very common in the early stages of a major stroke, the nursing staff performed a water swallow test. This was normal.

Mrs A was able to eat and drink. Within the next couple of days her blood pressure gradually came down and speech returned to normal.

An assessment was carried out by the physiotherapist and the occupational therapist and a programme of rehabilitation commenced.

The right side had been affected and she was right handed. The occupational therapist assisted with dressing practice; at first this uses strategies to overcome the loss of the use of one side. Someone at this stage may have to change the type of clothing normally worn to clothes that are easier to put on (fewer zips and buttons and shoes that slip on). Further occupational work would include bathroom and kitchen assessments.

Physiotherapy looked at movement and tone. Mrs A was able to walk with the assistance of two people, but as her arm had little movement, extra care had to be taken over 'where it was'. The shoulder can be prone to damage if the arm is not carefully positioned and protected.

Mrs A made good progress with her therapies. As she had stairs at home, practising in the safety of the gym was important. A visit was arranged by the occupational therapist to visit Mrs A at home to see how she would function in her own environment. Her husband was there, there was a banister on the stair, she was able to get on and off the toilet by herself and there was a walk-in shower. The occupational therapist was happy that there were no safety issues and it was decided that Mrs A could go home and then attend the local day hospital for a further 6 weeks to receive out-patient therapy.

All the medications she had been on previously were restarted apart from the Prempak-C (combined hormone replacement therapy is not generally recommended after an ischaemic stroke) and in addition she was started on dipyridamole MR (Persantin) (which when combined with aspirin may confer additional benefits) and a statin to lower the cholesterol level as well as receiving dietary advice.

She had been in hospital for 3 weeks. After discharge home she continued to do the exercises recommended and made a steady recovery.

Case 2

Mrs B is a 78-year-old who lives in sheltered housing. She was found collapsed by her warden and there was an obvious right-sided weakness. The warden called for an ambulance and Mrs B was admitted to hospital.

She had had mobility problems due to osteoarthritis and osteoporosis and walked with a stick and had a home help once a week.

Her risk factors for stroke were:

- Her age.
- Hypertension, which was being treated with doxazosin and perindopril.

When Mrs B was examined at the hospital she had a dense, right-sided weakness, with increased tone in her leg, slurred speech and a right homonymous hemianopia, and she appeared confused.

Routine tests

- Blood pressure was high at 245/116. This is very high at this stage but no treatment was given initially (generally therapy to lower blood pressure in the acute phase of stroke is not recommended as it may compromise blood flow to the brain).
- Pulse was 78 regular and normal.
- An ECG (tracing of the heart) was normal.
- CT scan showed a bleed in the brain in an area called the left basal ganglia.
- Swallow assessment was normal.

Assessments were carried out by the physiotherapist, the occupational therapist and the speech and language therapist. She received a therapy programme for her slurred speech and exercises to help this recover within 2 weeks. A rehabilitation programme from physiotherapy and occupational therapy was designed. Mrs B stuck to this programme and made good progress. After 2 weeks, she was transferred to a rehabilitation ward in an elderly medicine hospital and with 2 weeks of further therapy was safely discharged home after a home visit by the therapists.

Before discharge, amlodipine was added to help control her blood pressure. She had had problems in the past with diuretic drugs causing incontinence and so they were avoided. Aspirin and other similar drugs had to be avoided after this stroke, which had been caused by a bleed.

Case 3

Mr C is a 59-year-old retired policeman, who works as a security officer. He awoke at 2 a.m. to go to the toilet and discovered that his right side was slightly weak, his speech was slurred and he had decreased sensation. He woke his wife who is an auxiliary nurse and she recognized the symptoms as being that of a stroke and dialled 999.

On examination at the hospital, Mr C had a mild weakness of the right side including face, some slurring of speech and mild word-finding problems. The right side also felt funny. Mr C had previously been fit and well. On further questioning he described an episode of a few weeks previously where he had felt a curtain come down over his left eye. This had lasted a few minutes only and he had thought nothing of it. This had been an episode of amaurosis fugax.

Risk factors

- Smoking (Mr C was a heavy smoker).
- Amaurosis fugax (not reported to medical personnel).

Routine tests

- Blood pressure was 110/66, pulse 58, temperature normal.
- ECG was normal.

- 24-Hour ECG was normal.
- Blood tests were all within normal limits. Fasting glucose was normal at 4.0 while cholesterol was 4.8 mmol/l.
- CT scan showed an infarct in the left middle cerebral artery area.
- Carotid Doppler scan showed a stenosis of the left internal carotid artery of 79%.

As well as the normal assessment and therapy programme, Mr C was referred to the vascular surgeons for assessment for suitability of the operation, carotid endarterectomy.

Mr C was young, had been fit and active, went to the gym regularly, still worked and drove a car, the stenosis was within the range to consider operating and he fulfilled the criteria. He had made a very good and quick recovery from his weakness.

Prior to going for the operation, Mr C was commenced on clopidogrel (since he had experienced a gastrointestinal upset with aspirin when he was younger) and a statin. He was also counselled about giving up smoking and supplied with the smoking helpline number and information on patches and chewing gum.

Mr C was also given information regarding driving.

He was discharged after 5 days with a date to return in 4 weeks for his operation.

He returned for the operation, which was successful, and was able to return to his work, driving and all his leisure activities within 2 months of the stroke. He has managed to stop smoking and is doing well.

Case 4

Mrs D was a 79-year-old war widow who was a retired nurse. While out shopping one morning she had difficulty counting the money from her purse and was unable to speak, noting word-finding difficulties. Her friends noticed a drooping of the right side of her mouth. She rested at home and within 2 hours she was completely back to normal. She reported to her GP who referred her to the clinic.

Risk factors

- Atrial fibrillation (episodic is a risk factor).

- Hypertension.
- Angina.
- Cholesterol above 3.5 mmol/l.

On close questioning she had noticed palpitations (feeling fast irregular heart beats) from time to time over the past year. She had a history of hypertension treated with bendrofluazide and angina treated with a long-acting nitrate.

Routine tests

- Examination was entirely normal. Blood pressure was 150/88 at clinic.
- Normal routine bloods, fasting glucose 5.6 mmol/l, cholesterol 6 mmol/l.
- 12-Lead ECG showed left ventricular hypertrophy and a 24-hour tape ECG showed several episodes of atrial fibrillation.
- CT scan and carotid duplex Doppler scans were both entirely normal.

After discussion of the risks and benefits of anticoagulation therapy with warfarin and securing the help of her general practitioner who would monitor her INR (internationalized normalized ratio for blood coagulation) regularly and felt confident to do so, she was commenced on warfarin. Blood pressure was reduced with an angiotensin receptor blocker (she had a dry cough with the ACE inhibitor) and diuretic combination and a statin was used to reduce cholesterol. She had no further events even 5 years later and continued to enjoy her walking and swimming leisure time.

Case 5

Mrs E had had diabetes controlled with insulin for 30 years. She was now 52. When she woke one day she noticed she had no movement in her left arm and left hand. She could not get out of bed. Her husband could not get her out either. They called the GP who looked in later that morning. There had been no improvement so he sent her in to hospital.

She had a strong family history of stroke and myocardial infarction. Her father had had a stroke at age 54 and died of myocardial infarction at age 58. Her mother died of a stroke at age 66.

Examination revealed a flaccid weakness of the left arm and leg and there was weakness of the left half of the face and tongue. The left palate was weak and she choked on a water swallow test of 5 ml sterile water. She also was noted to have sensory inattention on the left side and an upper quadrant partial homonymous hemianopia. Blood pressure was 145/88 and her glucose on admission was 12 mmol/l. Her cholesterol was 7 mmol/l.

ECG showed some ischaemic changes. CT scan showed a large infarct in the middle cerebral artery territory on the right. Duplex Doppler scan of the carotid showed a complete occlusion of the right internal carotid artery.

Since she had swallowing difficulties, she was managed with nil by mouth overnight and her glucose controlled with a sliding scale insulin regimen and intravenous fluids. Next morning the speech and language therapist advised a nasogastric tube for feeding and this continued for a fortnight. Since swallowing was still a problem at this time, a PEG (percutaneous endoscopically placed gastrostomy) tube was inserted and this was cosmetically more acceptable to the patient and her family and allowed feeding overnight.

The physiotherapist and occupational therapist devised a rehabilitation plan and she regained sitting balance in a week and began standing in 2 weeks. She was transferred to a younger persons' specialist rehabilitation ward and continued to improve for a further 4 months. The sensory inattention was a challenge to the rehabilitation team but they had seen this before and had devised strategies to help promote recovery. She was then allowed home for several weekend breaks before her final discharge. She needed an attendant-propelled wheelchair to help mobility when she went outside for long distances but had regained the power to walk indoors and short distances outdoors. She had initial difficulties dressing but these problems had largely been resolved by her discharge. She continued to make progress at home.

Medications were used to control her blood pressure, using ACE inhibitors and calcium antagonists. She had aspirin and dipyridamole MR combination antiplatelet therapy and a statin helped reduce her cholesterol. Attention to diet and insulin helped her glucose control. She had a period of depression during the recovery period but this responded to antidepressant medication and reassuring words from the staff (it had taken a very long time and a lot of hard work from the patient to achieve independence once again).

These are simply examples of patients' strokes and their recovery. You may have more stories you could tell us about.

APPENDIX

Calculate your own stroke risk

Preventing stroke can be simple and Royal & Sun Alliance and the Stroke Foundation of New Zealand have developed a risk table which you can use to modify your risk of stroke.

Risk table for stroke

Risk factors	0	1	2	3	Current Score 1	Reduced Score 2
Smoked	Never smoked or quit more than 5 years ago	Quit after smoking for less than 5 years	Current smoker, less than 20/day	Current smoker, more than 20/day		
Exercise	1 hour energetic activity at least 3 times/week	Very active once or twice a week	Moderately active once or twice a week	Very little physical activity		
Diabetes	None known	–	Family history	Diabetic		
Blood pressure	Normal	Mild high blood pressure	Moderate high blood pressure	Severe high blood pressure		
Age	0–44	45–64	65–74	75+		
Alcohol (male)	0–2 standard drinks/day	Up to 4 drinks/day	More than 4 drinks/day 2 or more days/week	More than 6 drinks/day 4 or more days/week		
Alcohol (female)	0–1 standard drinks/day	Up to 2 drinks/day	More than 2 drinks/day 2 or more days/week	More than 4 drinks/day 4 or more days/week		
Weight	About average for height	Slightly overweight	Moderately over weight	Obese		
Family history	No strokes known	A relative has had a stroke	A relative has had a stroke while younger than 65	Several relatives have suffered from a stroke		
Cholesterol	Below average	Average	Moderately raised	Severely raised		
				Total		

Add up your total score. The lower your score, the better. The higher your score, the greater your risk of having a stroke. An approximate guide to the risk is: 0–4, very low risk; 5–9, moderate risk; 10–13, high risk; 14+, very high risk. See your doctor if you are concerned about your risk of stroke or want more information.

Reproduced with permission from Stroke Foundation of NZ Inc., PO Box 12482, Wellington, NZ. Tel: 04 472 8099; Fax: 04 472 7019; e-mail: strokenz@stroke.org.nz; Freephone: 0800 STROKE 0800 787 653.

Useful websites

- The Stroke Association: http://www.stroke.org.uk
- Chest, Heart & Stroke Scotland: http://www.chss.org.uk
- Stroke Information Directory: http://www.stroke-info.com
- Dundee Stroke Studies Centre: http://www.dundee.ac.uk/medicine/stroke/sites.html
- The Stroke Foundation of New Zealand: http://www.stroke.org.nz/index.html

Societies and associations

Stroke Association

Stroke House, 123–127 Whitecross Street, London EC1Y 8JJ
Tel: 020 7566 0300 Fax: 020 7490 2686 Helpline: 0845 30 33 100
Email: info@stroke.org.uk Website: www.stroke.org.uk
Information and advice about stroke illness

Chest, Heart & Stroke Scotland

65 North Castle Street, Edinburgh EH2 3LT
Tel: 0131 225 6963 Advice line: 0845 077 6000
(Mon–Fri 9.30am–12.30pm; 1.30pm–4pm) Fax: 0131 220 6313
Email:adviceline@chss.org.uk Website: www.chss.org.uk
Advice and local groups for stroke survivors in Scotland. Also funds research into stroke

Northern Ireland Chest, Heart & Stroke Association

21 Dublin Road, Belfast BT2 7HB
Tel: 028 9032 0184 Fax: 028 9033 3487 Advice Helpline: 084 077 6000 Website: www.nichsa.com
Advice and support for stroke survivors in Northern Ireland

Different strokes

162 High Street, Watford, Herts WD1 2EG
Tel: 01923 240615 Fax: 01923 240624 Email: info@differentstrokes.co.uk
Website: www.differentstrokes.co.uk
Support for younger people with stroke

Other helpful addresses

Action on Smoking and Health (ASH)

102 Clifton Street, London EC2A 4HW
Tel: 020 7739 5902 Website: www.ash.org.uk
Information on how smoking affects medical conditions and advice on stopping

Alzheimer's Society

Gordon House, 10 Greencoat Place, London SW1P 1PH
Tel: 020 7306 0606 Fax: 020 7306 0808 Helpline: 0845 3000 336
(Mon–Fri 8am–6.30pm) Website: www.alzheimers.org.uk
The main charity providing information and support for people with Alzheimer's disease and their carers

Association of Charity Officers

Beechwood House, Wyllyotts Close, Potters Bar, Herts EN6 2HN
Tel: 01707 651777 Fax: 01707 660477
Advice about charities that might be able to help you

Age Concern England

1268 London Road, London SW16 4ER
Tel: 020 8765 7200 Fax: 020 8765 7211 Information line: 0800 009966
Website: www.ageconcern.org.uk
Provides advice on a range of subjects for older people

Age Concern Scotland

Leonard Small House, 113 Rose Street, Edinburgh EH2 3DT
Tel: 0131 220 3345 Fax: 0131 220 2779 Freephone: 0800 00 99 66
(7am–7pm, 7 days a week) E-mail: enquiries@acscot.org.uk Website: www.ageconcernscotland.org.uk

Association of Independent Care Advisers

58 Southwick Street, Southwick BN42 4TJ
Tel: 01483 203066 Fax: 01483 202535 Website: www.aica.org.uk
Information and advaice about care options for people with learning or physical disabilities

Benefits Enquiry Line (BEL)

Benefit Enquiry Line, Victoria House, 9th Floor, Ormskirk Road, Preston, Lancashire, PR1 2QP
Tel: 0800 88 22 00 Fax: 01772 23 89 53 (Mon–Fri 8.30am–6.30pm; Sat 9am–1pm); for help in filling in claim forms: 0800 441144
Or see the telephone directory for your local office
Website: www.dwp.gov.uk/lifeevent/benefits/index.htm
For information on state benefits for people with disabilities and their carers

British Acupuncture Council

63 Jeddo Road, London W12 9HQ
Tel: 020 8735 0400 Fax: 020 8735 0404 Website: www.acupuncture.org.uk
Acupuncture practitioners' regulatory authority

British Association for Counselling

1 Regent Place, Rugby, Warwickshire CV21 2PJ
Tel: 0870 443 5252 Fax: 0870 443 5160
Website: www.counselling.co.uk
Can help with finding counselling services in your area

British Heart Foundation

14 Fitzhardinge Street, London W1H 4DH
Tel: 020 7935 0185 Fax: 020 7486 5820 Website: www.bhf.org.uk
A charity funding research into heart disease, and providing help and advice

British Lung Foundation

78 Hatton Garden, London EC1N 8LD
Tel: 020 7831 5831 Fax: 020 7831 5832 Website: www.lunguk.org
A charity funding research into breathing diseases, and providing help and advice

British Red Cross

9 Grosvenor Crescent, London SW1X 7EJ
Tel: 020 7235 5454 Fax: 020 7245 6315 Website: www.redcross.org.uk
Has home aids available for hire

Calibre Cassette Library

New Road, Weston Turville, Aylesbury, Buckingham HP22 5XQ
Tel: 01296 432339 Fax: 01296 392599 Website: www.calibre.org.uk
Audio cassette library for visually impaired people

Carers National Association (CAN)

20–25 Glasshouse Yard, London EC1A 4JT
Tel: 020 7490 8818 Fax: 020 7490 8824 Carersline – advice line for carers at the cost of a local call: 0345 573 369
Advice and support for carers

Carers National Association Scotland

91 Mitchell Street, Glasgow G1 3LN
Tel: 0141 221 9141 CarersLine: 0345 573 369

Child Poverty Action Group

94 White Lion Street, London N1 9PF
Website: www.cpag.org.uk
Promotes action for the relief, directly or indirectly, of poverty among children and families with children

Church of Scotland

Board of Social Responsibility, Charis House, 47 Milton Road East, Edinburgh EH15 2SR
Tel: 0131 657 2000 Website: www.churchofscotland.org.uk
Scotland's largest voluntary sector social work agency

Connect (Communication Disability Network)

16–18 Marshalsea Road, London SE1 1HL
Tel: 020 7367 0840 Fax: 020 7347 0841 Email: info@ukconnect.org
Website: www.ukconnect.org
Help for people with communication problems

Continence Foundation

307 Hatton Square, 16 Baldwins Gardens, London EC1N 7RJ
Tel: 0845 345 0165 (Mon–Fri, 9:30am–12:30pm)
Website: www.continence-foundation.org.uk
For advice, and a continence adviser near you. Also has leaflets on incontinence

Counsel and Care

Lower Gound Floor, Twyman House, 16 Bonny Street, London NW1 9PG
Tel: 020 7241 8555 Helpline: 0845 300 7585 (Mon–Fri, 10am–1pm)
Website: www.counselandcare.org.uk
For advice on remaining at home or about care homes

Court of Protection

Public Trust Office Protection Division, Stewart House, 24 Kingsway, London WC2B 6JX
Tel: 020 7664 7000 (Mon–Fri, 9am–5pm) Fax: 020 7664 7705 Website: www.publictrust.gov.uk
If you need to take over the affairs of someone who is mentally incapable (in England and Wales)

Crossroads – Caring for Carers

10 Regent Place, Rugby, Warwickshire CV21 2PN
Tel: 0845 450 0350 Fax: 01788 565498 Website: www.crossroads.org.uk
Can provide a paid, trained person to offer respite care in the home

CRUSE – Bereavement Care

126 Sheen Road, Richmond, Surrey TW9 1UR
Tel: (helpline) 0870 167 1677
Helpline email: helpline@crusebereavementcare.org.uk
Website: www.crusebereavementcare.org.uk
Bereavement advice and support

Department for Work and Pensions (DWP)

Department for Work and Pensions, Correspondence Unit, Room 540, The Adelphi, 1–11 John Adam Street, London WC2N 6HT
Tel: 020 7712 2171 (Mon–Fri, 9am–5pm) Tel: 0870 000 2288 Fax: 020 7712 2386 Website: www.dwp.gov.uk
Offers help to disabled for employment and advice pack on disability

DIAL UK (Disablement Information and Advice Lines)

St Catherine's, Tickhill Road, Doncaster DN4 8QN
Tel: 01302 310123 Fax: 01302 310404 Website: www.dialuk.org.uk
Information and advice for people with disabilities, including a network of 140 local centres

Disability Alliance

1st Floor, East Universal House, 88–94 Wentworth Street, London E1 7SA
Tel: 020 7247 8776 Fax 020 7247 8765
Website: www.disabilityalliance.org
Information on disability welfare benefits

Disability Information trust

Mary Marlborough Centre, Nuffield Orthopaedic Centre, Headington, Oxford OX3 7LD
Tel: 01865 227592
Website: www.abilityonline.org.uk/disability information trust.htm
Assesses and tests disability equipment on the market and publishes findings

Disability Law Service

39–45 Cavell Street, London E1 2BP
Tel: 020 7791 9800 Textphone: 020 7791 9801 Fax: 020 7791 9802
Website: www.abilityonline.org.uk/.disability law service.htm
Free legal advice for disabled people and their carers and families

Disabled Drivers Association

National HQ, Ashwellthorpe, Norwich, Norfolk NR16 1EX
Tel: 0870 770 3333 Fax: 01508 488173 Website: www.dda.org.uk
Information and advice for disabled drivers

Disabled Drivers' Motor Club

Cottingham Way, Thrapston, Northants NN14 4PL
Tel: 01832 734724 Fax: 01832 733816 Website: www.ddmc.org.uk
Information and advice about mobility problems for disabled people

Disabled Living Centres Council

Redbank House, 4 St Chad's Street, Manchester M8 8QA
Tel: 0161 834 1044 Fax: 0161 835 3591 Website: www.dlcc.org.uk
For the Disability Living Centre nearest you, where you can see aids and equipment

Disabled Living Foundation

380–384 Harrow Road, London W9 2HU
Tel: 020 7289 6111 Helpline: 0870 130 9177 Website: www.dlf.org.uk
For information about equipment to help you cope with a disability

Disablement Income Group (DIG)

Unit 5, Archway Business Centre, 19–23 Wedmore Street, London N19 4RZ
Tel: 020 7263 3981
Working to improve the financial circumstances of disabled people

Disablement Income Group Scotland (DIG)

5 Quayside Street, Edinburgh EH6 6EJ
Tel: 0131 555 2811
Runs a free benefits advisory and advocacy service

Discern

Suite 6, Clarendon Chambers, Clarendon St, Nottingham NG1 5LN
Tel: 0115 947 4147 Website: www.discerncounselling.org.uk
A charity to help people with physical disability or learning difficulties who experience problems with sex or personal relationships

Elderly Accommodation Counsel

3rd Floor, 89 Albert Embankment, London SE1 7TP
Tel: 020 7820 1343 Fax: 020 7820 3970 Website: www.housingcare.org
Information about all forms of accommodation for older people

Free Prescriptions Advice Line

Tel: 0800 9177 711 (Mon–Fri 8am–6pm; Sat & Sun 10am–4pm)
Advice on entitlement to free dental and optical care and eyesight tests

Greater London Association for Disabled People (GLAD)

336 Brixton Road, London SW9 7AA
Tel: 020 7346 5800 Fax: 020 7346 5810 Website: www.glad.org.uk
Information for disabled Londoners

Headway (The Brain Injury Association)

4 King Edward Court, King Edward Street, Nottingham NG1 1EW
Tel: 0115 924 0800 Fax: 0115 958 4446 Helpline: 0115 924 0800
Website: www.headway.org.uk
Provides information, support and services to people who have suffered a head injury, their family and carers

Help the Aged

England: 207–221 Pentonville Road, London N1 9UZ
Tel: 020 7278 1114 Fax: 020 7278 1116 Email: info@helptheaged.org.uk
Scotland: 11 Granton Square, Edinburgh EH5 1HX
Tel: 0131 551 6331 Fax: 0131 551 5415 Email: infoscot@helptheaged
Ireland: Ascot House, 24–30 Shaftesbury Square, Belfast BT2 7DB
Tel: 02890 230 666 Fax: 02890 248 183 Email: infoni@helptheaged.org.uk
Wales: Room 123, CSV House, Williams Way, Cardiff CF10 5DY
Tel: 02920 415 711 Fax: 02920 415 712
Email: infocymru@helptheaged.org.uk Website: www.helptheaged.org.uk
Advice and support for older people and carers

Holiday Care

2nd Floor, Imperial Buildings, Victoria Road, Horley, Surrey RH6 7PZ
Information: 0845 124 9971 Website: www.holidaycare.org.uk
Information and advice about holidays, travel or respite care for older or disabled people and carers

Impotence Association

PO Box 10296, London SW17 9WH
Tel: 020 8767 7791 Website: www.impotence.org.uk
Help and advice on sexual problems

Independent Living (1993) Fund

PO Box 183, Nottingham NG8 3RD
Tel: 0115 942 8191 Fax: 0115 929 3156 Email: Funds@ilf.org.uk or Csmanager@ilf.org.uk
May fund very severely disabled people between 16 and 65 years of age to buy in extra care

Jewish Care

Stuart Young House, 221 Golders Green Road, London NW11 9DQ
Tel: 020 8922 2000 Email: info@jcare.org Website: www.jewishcare.org
Social care, personal support and residential homes for Jewish people

John Groom's

45/50 Scrutton Street, London EC2A 4XQ
Tel: 020 7452 2000 Fax: 020 7452 2001 Website: www.johngrooms.org.uk
A christian charity providing residential, respite and holiday accommodation

Leonard Cheshire

30 Millbank, London SW1P 4QD
Tel: 020 7802 8200 Fax: 020 7802 8250 Email: info@london.leonard-cheshire.org.uk Website: www.leonard-cheshire.org
Residential homes and home care attendants for disabled people and Workability scheme for job finding

Mobility Advice and Vehicle Information Service (MAVIS)

Department of Transport, O Wing, MacAdam Avenue, Old Wokingham Road, Crowthorpe, Berkshire RG45 6XD
Tel: 01344 661000 Fax: 01344 661066 Email: mavis@dft.gsi.gov.uk
Website: www.mobility-unit.dft.gov.uk
Advice on car adaptations and transport for disabled people

Motability

Goodman House, Station Approach, Harlow, Essex CM20 2ET
Tel: 01279 635666 Fax: 01279 632000 Website: www.motability.co.uk
Advice and help about cars, scooters and wheelchairs for disabled people

National Association of Bereavement Services

2 Plough Yard, London EC2A
Tel: 020 7247 1080 Tel: 020 7247 0617 Fax: 020 7247 0617
Information about bereavement and loss counselling in your area (written enquires only)

National Association of Citizens Advice Bureaux

115–123 Pentonville Road, London N1 9LZ
Tel: 020 7833 2181 Fax: 020 7833 4371
Website: www.citizensadvice.org.uk
For advice on legal, financial and consumer matters. Good general source of information. See you telephone book for the one in your area

National Association of Councils for Voluntary Service

3rd Floor, Arundel Court, 177 Arundel Street, Sheffield S1 2NU
Tel: 0114 278 6636 Fax: 0114 278 7004 Website: www.nacvs.org.uk
Promotes and supports the work of councils for voluntary service throughout England

National Association of Funeral Directors

618 Warwick Road, Solihull, Birmingham B91 1AA
Tel: 0121 711 1343 Fax: 0121 711 1351
Offers a code of conduct and a simple service for a basic funeral

National Council for Voluntary Organisations (NCVO)

Regents Wharf, 8 All Saints Street, London N1 9RL
Tel: 020 7713 6161 Fax: 020 7713 6300 Website: www.ncvo-vol.org.uk
Information on local voluntary organisations that may be able to provide help

National Health Service Helpline

England and Wales: NHS Direct: 0845 4647 NHS helpline: 0800 22 44 88
NHS Direct www.nhsdirect.nhs.uk
Scotland: 0800 22 44 88
Speak to a nurse for some common-sense advice about your health

Pensions Advisory Service

11 Belgrave Road, London SW1V 1RB
National helpline: 0845 601 2923 Website: www.opas.org.uk
For queries and problems to do with occupational pensions

Phab

Summit House, Wandle Road, Croydon, Surrey CR0 1DF
Tel: 020 8667 9443 Fax: 020 8681 1399 email: info@phabengland.org.uk
Website: www.phabengland.org.uk
Works to promote integration between disabled and non-disabled people on equal terms

Princess Royal Trust for Carers

London Office: 142 Minories, London EC3N 1LB
Tel: 020 7480 7788 Fax 020 7481 4729 Email: info@carers.org
Northern Office: Suite 4, Oak House, High Street, Chorley PR7 1DW
Tel: 01257 234070 Fax: 01257 234105 Email: infochorley@carers.org
Glasgow Office: Campbell House, 215 West Campbell Street, Glasgow G2 4TT
Tel: 0141 221 5066 Fax 0141 221 4623 Email: infoscotland@carers.org
Website: www.carers.org
Provides information, support and practical help for carers; your phone book may list a local branch

Quit

Victory House, 170 Tottenham Court Road, London W1P 0HA
Tel: 020 7388 5775 Fax: 020 7388 5995 Website: www.quit.org.uk
National charity helping smokers to stop smoking; see Quitline, below

Quitline (Smokeline in Scotland)

England: 0800 00 22 00 (12–9pm 7 days a week)
N Ireland: 02890 663281
Scotland: 0800 84 84 84 (noon–midnight 7 days a week)
Wales: 0345 697 500
Hor help and advice on giving up smoking

RADAR (Royal Association for Disability and Rehabilitation)

12 City Forum, 250 City Road, London EC1V 8AF
Tel: 020 7250 3222 Fax: 020 7250 0212 Website: www.radar.org.uk
General information about disability

Registered Nursing Homes Association

15 Highfield Road, Edgbaston, Birmingham B15 3DU
Tel: 0121 454 2511 Freephone: 0800 074 0194 Fax: 0121 454 9032
Website: www.rnha.co.uk
Information about registered nursing homes in your area

Rehab Scotland

Head Office, 1650 London Road, Glasgow G31 4QF
Tel: 0141 554 8822 Email: headoffice@rehab-scotland.co.uk
Website: www.rehab.ie/scotland/index.htm
Help in Scotland for those whose lives have been shattered by disability

Relate (formerly National Marriage Guidance Council)

Herbert Gray College, Little Church Street, Rugby, Warwickshire CV212 3AP
Tel: 01788 573241 or (lo-call) 0845 456 1310 Website: www.relate.org.uk
Counselling and help with difficult relationships

Remploy

415 Edgware Road, London NW2 6LR
Tel: 0800 138 7656 Fax 0800 138 7657 Website: www.remploy.co.uk
Advice about returning to work

Scottish Association for Mental Health

Cumbrae House, 15 Carlton Court, Glasgow G5 9JP
Tel: 0141 568 7000 Fax: 0141 568 7001 Website: www.samh.org.uk
Information about services in Scotland for people with mental health problems

Scottish Council for Voluntary Organisations

The Mansfield, Traquair Centre, 15 Mansfield Place, Edinburgh EH3 6BB
Tel: 0131 556 3882 Fax: 0131 556 0279 Website: www.scvo.org.uk
For information about voluntary organisations in Scotland

Shaftesbury Housing Group

Shaftesbury House, 87 East Street, Epsom, Surrey KT17 1DT
Tel: 01372 727252 Website: www.shaftesburyhousing.org.uk
Sheltered housing for older people in some areas

Shaw Trust

Shaw House, Epsom Square, White Horse Business Park, Trowbridge, Wilts BA14 0XJ
Tel: 01225 716350 Fax: 01225 716334 Website: www.shaw-trust.org.uk
Advice to help people with disabilities return to work

Soldiers, Sailors and Airmen Family Association (SSAFA)

19 Queen Elizabeth Street, London SE1 2LP
Tel: 020 7403 8783 Email: info@ssafa.org.uk Website: www.ssafa.org.uk
Help for service or ex-service people and their families

Speakability (formerly Action for Dysphasic Adults)

1 Royal Street, London SE1 7LN
Tel: 020 7261 9572 Fax: 020 7928 9542 Helpline: 080 8808 9572 (Mon–Fri 10am–4pm) Website: www.speakability.org.uk
Help for adults with language problems (dysphasia). Has literature and local support groups

SPOD (Association to Aid the Sexual and Personal Relationships of People with a Disability)

286 Camden Road, London N7 0BJ
Tel: 020 7607 8851 Fax 020 7700 0236 Email: info@spod-uk.org Website: www.spod-uk.org
Help with sexual problems

Tripscope
The Vassal Centre, Gill Avenue, Bristol BS16 2QQ
Tel: 0117 939 7782 Fax: 0117 939 7736 Helpline: 08457 58 56 41 Website: www.tripscope.org.uk
Information and advice about travel and transport for disabled and older people and their carers

UK Home Care Association (UKHCA)
42B Banstead Road, Carshalton Beeches, Surrey SM5 3NW
Tel: 020 8288 1551 Fax: 020 8288 1550 Website: www.ukhca.co.uk
Information about member organisations providing home care in your area

Wales Council for Voluntary Action
Llys Ifor, Crescent Road, Caerphilly, Mid Glamorgan CF83 1XL
Tel: 02920 855100 Fax: 02920 855101 Website: www.wcva.org.uk
Information about voluntary groups in Wales

Women's Royal Voluntary Service (WRVS)
Milton Hill House, Milton Hill, Abingdon, Oxon OX13 6AF
Tel: 01235 442900 Fax: 01235 861166 Email: enquiries@wrvs.org.uk
Website: www.wrvs.org.uk
Provides meals-on-wheels and other services in certain areas

Useful Publications

- *Care after Stroke: Information for patients and their carers*
  by Marcia Kelson and Penny Irwin (based on the NHS Executive's *National Clinical Guidelines for Stroke*), Royal College of Physicians, London (2000).
- *Caring for Someone who has had a Stroke*
  by Philip Coyne with Penny Mares, Age Concern England, London (1995).
- *A Guide to Grants for Individuals in Need*
  edited by S Harland, Directory of Social Change, London (1998/9).

- *Stroke at your Fingertips*
  by Anthony Rudd, Penny Irwin, Bridget Penhale, Class, London (2000).
- *My Year Off*
  by Robert McCrum, Picador, London (1998). Compelling story of survival after stroke.

INDEX

Note: page numbers in *italics* refer to figures and tables

ACE inhibitors 54, 65
acupuncture 50
aerobic capacity 51
age 8
aids 55
alcohol consumption 10, 13, 38, 42
  safe limits 51
amaurosis fugax 24, 62
amlopidine 62
aneurysm formation 7
angina 17–18, 64
  family history 38
angioplasty 38
antibiotics 44, 47
anticoagulant drugs 44, 53, 64
anticonvulsant drugs 49
antidepressants 49, 66
antihypertensive drugs 44
antiplatelet drugs 44, 53, 65
  see also aspirin; clopidogrel; dipyridamole
anxiety *21*, 25, 50
aphasia *21*, 22–3, 37
arteries
  blocked/burst *4*, 7
  hardening 13, 15
aspirin 44, 48, 53
  avoidance 62
  case studies 59, 61, 65
associations for support/help 68–9
atherosclerosis *4*, 13, 15
  cholesterol-lowering drugs 44
atorvastatin 53

atrial fibrillation 17, 44, 53
attitude, positive 55

balance loss *21*, 26, 37
bathroom assessment 60
bendrofluazide 54
binge drinking 10, 51
bladder control *21*, 25
blood circulation 51
blood clots 13, 48
  'dissolving' 43
  echocardiogram 34
  heart disease 17–18
  high red blood cell count 16
  prevention 44, 53
  smoking 9, 43
blood clotting disorders 7
  see also clotting factors
blood pressure
  24-hour monitoring 35
  control 14
  ethnic groups 9
  increase 52
  lowering 39, 40, 44, 51, 54, 55
blood pressure, high 12, 13–14, 15
  alcohol consumption 10, 42
  case study 64
  diabetes 17
  family history 38
  heart disease risk 18
  obesity/overweight 17, 40, 51
  stress 42, 52
  treatment 39, 40, 44, 51, 54, 55
blood tests 27

85

blood vessels 13, 15
  blocked *4, 7*
  burst *4*, 7, 13
body mass index (BMI) 10, *11*
bowels
  control *21*, 25
  function 49
brain
  scans 28, *29–32*, 33
  structure 19, *20*, 21
brainstem *20*, 21
  haemorrhage *31*
bronchitis 43
bupropion 10
bypass grafts 38

calcium antagonists 65
carbohydrates 41
  refined 40
carers 70
  communication problems 23
carotid angioplasty 44
carotid arteries
  disease 13, 15–16
  duplex Doppler 33
  magnetic resonance angiography *34*, 35
  occlusion 65
carotid endarterectomy 16, 44, 63
case studies 59–66
cerebellar infarct *33*
cerebellum *20*, 21
  MRI scan *33*
cerebral cortex 19, *20*
cerebral haemorrhage 3, *4, 5*
  CT scan *30*
  MRI scan *32*
cerebral infarct 3, *4*, 6
  CT scan *28, 29*
  MRI scan *31–2*
cerebrospinal fluid (CSF) 35–6
chiropodists 46

cholesterol, 'good' 12, 41
cholesterol, high level 13, 14–15, 41
  diabetes 17
  family history 38
  heart disease risk 18
  lowering 44, 51, 53, 55, 61
  obesity 17
  smoking 43
cholesterol-lowering drugs 44
  see also statins
clopidogrel 44, 53, 63
clothing 60
clotting factors
  reduction 44
  tests 36
communication problems *21*, 23
complementary therapies 50
complications 47–50
compression stockings 48
computed tomography (CT) 3, *5, 6*, 28, *29–31*, 65
concentration, loss of 56
confusion 25
congestive heart failure 18
constipation 49
consultation 37–8
control taking 52
coordination loss *21*, 26, 37
coronary artery disease 12
cough reflex 47
counselling 57, 63, 69
Coversyl, *see* perindopril

dairy products 41
dementia 56
  multi-infarct 24
depression *21*, 25, 49
  management 52, 66
diabetes 16–17, 42
  atherosclerosis risk 15
  blood glucose control 54

case studies 59, 64
family history 38
obesity 17
diagnosis of stroke 27–8, *29–32*, 33–6
diastolic blood pressure 14
diet 10, 12, 13
   advice 61
   changes 39–40
   diabetes 54, 66
   low-fat 51
dieticians 46
dipyridamole 44, 53, 61, 65
Discern 57, 69
district nursing services 46
diuretics 54, 64
dizziness 26, 37
driving 49, 56–7, 63
duplex Doppler scan 33, 65
DVLA (Driver and Vehicle Licensing Agency) 49, 56–7
dysarthria *21*, 22, 37
dysphasia *21*, 22–3, 37

echocardiography (ECG) 33–4, 65
embolism 24, *32*
   pulmonary 48
emotional control loss *21*, 24, 49–50
epilepsy 49
ethnic groups 9
exercise 12, 13, 39, 40
   after stroke 55–6, 64
   avoiding falls 50
   isometric 52
   stroke prevention 51–2
   weight loss 51

falls 50
family history 9, 38, 65
fat, body 40
   see also obesity; overweight; weight, loss

fat, dietary 41–2
   animal 13, 39, 40, 41
   saturated 41, 42
fatigue *21*, 25, 55
feeding problems *21*, 23
feelings, sharing 52, 57
fibre intake 40, 41, 49
fish, oily 41
fluvastatin 53
fractures 50
fruit and vegetables 13, 39, 40, 41
frustration *21*, 24

gadgets 55
gender 8
glucose, blood levels 40, 42
   control 54, 66

haemorrhagic stroke 3, *4, 5*
   causes *4*, 7
   ethnic groups 9
   incidence 7
headache, severe 26, 37
health, general 12–13
heart attacks 17–18
   family history 38
   smoking 43
heart disease
   blood clots 17–18
   obesity 17
   risk factors 18
heart valve disease 17
hemianopia 24
   homonymous 61, 65
heparin 48
high density lipoprotein (HDL) 12, 15
home helps 46
hormone replacement therapy 59, 61
hypertension *see* blood pressure, high

ibuprofen 49

87

incontinence *21*, 25, 48
indapamide 54
infections 15, 44
   chest 47
   urinary 48
insulin 12, 54, 66
intracerebral haemorrhage *4*
ischaemic heart disease 13, 17–18
ischaemic stroke 3, *4*
   aspirin 44
   causes *4*, 7
   heart disease 17–18
   incidence 7

joint problems 48–9

kitchen assessment 60

left ventricular hypertrophy 18
lifestyle factors 7, 9–10, *11*, 12–18, 38
   treatments 39, 50–3
lipid-lowering therapy 15, 54
low density lipoprotein (LDL) 15
lumbar puncture 35–6
lung cancer 43

magnetic resonance angiography (MRA) *34*, 35
magnetic resonance imaging (MRI) 28, *31–3*
meals on wheels 46
medical examination 27–8, *29–32*, 33–6
medical history 38
medication 38, 53–4
   diabetes 42
meditation 42, 52
memory loss *21*, 24, 56
mini-stroke *see* transient ischaemic attacks (TIAs)
mitral stenosis 17

mobilization 48, 65
monounsaturated fats 41
mood changes *21*, 24–5, 49–50
morphine-related drugs 49
multi-infarct dementia 24
muscle paralysis *21*, 47
myocardial infarction 18, 65

nasogastric feeding 23, 65
NHS Helpline 69
nicotine replacement 10, 43, 50
non-steroidal anti-inflammatory drugs (NSAIDs) 49
numbness *21*, 25
nursing 48
   district 46

obesity 10, 12, 17, 48
   see also overweight
occupational therapy 45–6, 48
   assessment 60, 62, 65
older people 8
omega-3 fats 41
oral contraceptives 12
oral hypoglycaemic drugs 54
osteoporosis 50
out-patient therapy 60
overweight 40, 51
   see also obesity

pain killers 49
paracetamol 44, 49
PEG (percutaneous endoscopically placed gastrostomy) tube 23, 65
perindopril 54
Persantin *see* dipyridamole
physical activity *see* exercise
physical inactivity 12
physiotherapy 45–6, 48
   activity plan 51
   assessment 60, 62, 65
platelets 53

plavix *see* clopidogrel
polyunsaturated fats 41
pressure sores 48
prevastatin 53
prevention of further strokes 50–4
pulmonary thromboembolism 48

quadrantanopia 24

ramipril 54
recovery 45–6, 47, 55
recurrence of stroke 47
red blood cell count 13, 16
rehabilitation 45–6, 50
  case study 60, 62, 65
relaxation 42, 52
rest 52
rheumatoid arthritis 15
risk factors for stroke 8–10, *11,* 12–18
  case studies 59, 61, 62
  modifiable 8, 9–10, *11,* 12–18, 39
  non-modifiable 8–9
  see also lifestyle factors

salt, dietary 13, 39, 40
seizures 49
sensation loss *21,* 37, 48, 59
  joint pain 49
sensory inattention *21,* 65
sexual relations 57, 69
shoulder pain 49
sight *see* vision, partial loss
signs of stroke 21, 25–6
simvastatin 53
skin problems 48
skull, surgery within 45
smoking 9–10, 13, 18, 43
  atherosclerosis risk 15
  case study 62
  heart disease risk 18
  high red blood cell count 16
  information for doctor 38

oral contraceptives 12
  stopping 43, 50, 54, 63, 70
social workers 46
societies for support/help 68–9
socioeconomic factors 18
speech and language therapists 23, 45–6
  assessment 62
speech problems *21,* 22–3, 25, 37
  case studies 61, 62, 63
statins 15, 53–4
  case studies 61, 63, 64, 65
stress 42, 52
stroke
  incidence 6
  previous 9, 13, 16
  risk 67
  severity 55
  types 3, *4–5,* 6
subarachnoid haemorrhage *4*
sugar intake 42
support services 52
  at home 46
survival after stroke 47
swallowing problems *21,* 23, 65
  chest infections 47
symptoms of stroke 21–5, 37
  timing 37
systolic blood pressure 14

tai chi 56
thrombolysis 25, 43
tiredness *21,* 25, 55
transient ischaemic attacks (TIAs) 6, 13, 16
  driving 56
  family history 9, 38
  treatments 39–46
    lifestyle 39–43
    medical 43–4
    rehabilitation 45–6
    surgical 44–5

89

ultrasound scan 33, 34, 65
undernourishment 48
understanding difficulties *21,* 22–3, 25

vegetables 49
  see also fruit and vegetables
vision, partial loss 24, 26, 37
visual field defects 24
vitamins 41

waist measurement 12
waist to hip ratio 10, 12
walking problems 26

warfarin 44, 53, 64
warning signs 25–6
weakness *21,* 25, 37
  case study 59, 61, 62, 65
websites 68
weight
  control 55
  loss 13, 39, 51
  see also obesity; overweight
weight-lifting 52

yoga 42, 52

Zyban *see* bupropion